The Old Farmer's Almanac Home Library

TRADITIONAL
HOME
REMEDIES

Time-Tested Methods
for Staying Well —
The Natural Way

Martha White
AND THE EDITORS OF
The Old Farmer's Almanac

OLD FARMER'S ALMANAC HOME LIBRARY

Series Editor: Sarah Elder Hale

Consulting Editor: Susan Peery

Copy Editor: Barbara Jatkola

Art Director: Karen Savary

Layout: Sheryl Fletcher

Cover Illustration: Sara Love

LIBRARY OF CONGRESS CATALOGING-IN-PUBLICATION DATA
White, Martha.
Traditional home remedies : time-tested methods
for staying well — the natural way / Martha White and the
editors of the Old farmer's almanac.p.   cm. —
(Old farmer's almanac home library)
ISBN 0-7835-4868-0
1. Herbs — Therapeutic use. 2. Traditional medicine.
3. Naturopathy. I. Old farmer's almanac. II. Title.
III. Series. RM666.H33W46   1997
615′.321 — dc21   96-52374 CIP

Distributed in the book trade by Time-Life Books, Inc.

TIME-LIFE BOOKS IS A DIVISION OF TIME LIFE INC.

TIME-LIFE CUSTOM PUBLISHING
Vice President and Publisher: Terry Newell
Associate Publisher: Teresa Hartnett
Vice President of Sales and Marketing: Neil Levin
Director of New Product Development: Quentin McAndrew
Director of Special Sales: Liz Ziehl
Director of Editorial Development: Jennifer Pearce

TIME-LIFE is a trademark of Time Warner Inc. U.S.A.

TRADITIONAL
HOME
REMEDIES

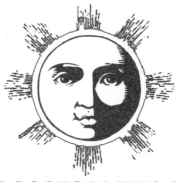

Contents

Foreword

OR WELL OVER 200 YEARS, READERS OF *THE OLD Farmer's Almanac* have been providing us with their home remedies. For the most part, these people may not know why a certain remedy works, but they have learned from their own experiences — and those of their parents and grandparents — that they do work.

Now, I have to admit that we receive a few remedies each year that stretch one's ability to believe. Cures for the common cold come to mind. We have dozens of remedies in our files involving items such as molasses, mustard packs, and pieces of flannel soaked in salve to wrap around one's neck. I believe these and other such remedies have merit, as they often help relieve cold symptoms.

However, I recall a letter from Illinois a few years back suggesting that the best cure for the common cold was to stand on one's head underwater. The writer swore it "works every time." Somehow, I don't think so. Another reader from Atlanta told us that his English aunt's severe case of the flu was instantly cured the moment most of her home in London was demolished by a V-2 missile during World War II. (Even he didn't go so far as to actually recommend it as a cure.)

Home remedies — the ones supported by many generations of successful use as well as the ones we can refer to only as "wacky" — have always been an integral part of *The Old Farmer's Almanac.* "Our purpose is to be useful," wrote the Almanac's founder, Robert B. Thomas, in his 1830 edition, "but with a pleasant degree of humor." If asked for our "mission statement" today, I wouldn't change a word.

What Is *The Old Farmer's Almanac?*

First of all, it's the oldest continuously published periodical in North America. It was established in 1792 by Robert B. Thomas, a Massachusetts schoolteacher whose name still appears on the familiar yellow cover, and it has appeared annually on the American scene every year since.

Like any publication legitimately calling itself an almanac, it is also, as such books were known in ancient times, a "calendar of the heavens." In other words, one of its primary duties is to provide the astronomical structure of the coming year on a daily basis.

Perhaps what *The Old Farmer's Almanac* is most of all, however, is a vast compendium of useful and entertaining information. Its major subjects include food, gardening, home remedies, history, and odd facts that you just won't find anywhere else. Oh, yes, it has weather forecasts, too. We can't forget those.

In the past decade, during which the circulation has skyrocketed to include some 9 million readers annually, the Almanac has added a feature section covering current consumer tastes and trends — from collectibles to fashions to health news to money-saving ideas to, well, just about everything going on in America today.

So even though the Almanac is old, it is also brand-new every year. And in addition to being America's oldest publication, perhaps it has become, over these many years, America's most loved publication as well.

JUDSON D. HALE, SR.
Editor-in-Chief
The Old Farmer's Almanac
(The 12th editor since 1792)

Introduction

*I*F YOU'VE EVER READ AN EARLY "RECEIPT" BOOK passed down through the generations, you've no doubt noticed that home remedies are interspersed with the custards and mincemeats and wedding cakes. You're apt to find the cure for croup right next to the batter pudding or the slippery elm cough drops next to the pickled cherries. Clearly, in earlier days, the pantry (or larder) and the medicine cabinet often were stocked from the same kitchen garden. Foodstuffs were both nutrition and good medicine, some preventive and some curative, but never disassociated in the way we tend to think of them today.

Now when we walk through our huge, modern supermarkets, most of us look at the wares as possible meals rather than as potential apothecary supplies. Similarly, our fields, woods, and gardens are more ornamental than functional. Even those of us who plant vegetables and herbs use them only to supplement our year-round stores of produce. For the most part, we've lost touch with foods as healing agents.

Increasingly, however, modern-day science has reinforced what our ancestors knew about apples, cranberries, chicken soup, vinegar, herbs, and countless other foods. Meanwhile, the new "miracle drugs" turn out to be derivatives or synthetic versions of age-old remedies. Cortisone mimics an ingredient in sarsaparilla (ginger ale and Coca-Cola were originally medicinal, too); digitoxin (used to treat cardiac conditions) comes from the foxglove plant, morphine from the opium poppy, and quinine from cinchona bark; and another coronary drug duplicates the effects of red clover. Even common aspirin is a synthesized version of salicin, obtained mainly from willow and poplar bark and many other herbal sources.

As we learn more about the foods and herbs that nurture our bodies and spirits, it becomes evident that some rudimentary herbal know-how, allowing us to concoct recipes and make bath preparations from our kitchen gardens, moves us toward a healthier, more independent, and more ecologically responsible way of life. For those of us without kitchen gardens, the health food store and local grocery do very nicely, once we know what we need. Far from being snake oil and quackery, home remedies are, for the most part, a simple matter of choosing a purposeful and healthful diet, knowing how to eat locally and seasonally, and recognizing that a few topical healing agents (such as aloe, garlic, onion, lavender oil, and witch hazel) should be part of any household's first aid kit and prevention program.

Educating ourselves about how to prevent and ease illness doesn't mean abandoning our trusted health practitioners but instead assisting them by taking better care of ourselves. Utilizing the healing benefits of a wide variety of foods and herbs is one way we can improve our well-being. Home remedies encourage us to be at home in our gardens and woods, to learn more about the foods we eat, and to slow down for a soothing cup of tea, a relaxing herb bath, or an invigorating spring tonic. Isn't it time we listened to our ancestors?

A Cautionary Note

Respect your ingredients and educate yourself about them. Be sure to use the part of the plant specified, whether flowers, stems, leaves, roots, or bark. Generally, if no part is noted, it is the aerial parts (leaves, stems, and flowers) that are used. Also consider your own particular sensitivities (which can be very different from those of someone else) and closely observe the results of any remedy. Keep in mind John Wesley's 18th-century note that "the medicine which cures one man will not always cure another of the same distemper. Nor will it cure the same man at all times. Therefore it [is] necessary to have a variety." See Chapter 8 for more cautionary advice and Appendix I for cautions related to specific plants.

Sources & Abbreviations

In the following pages, we refer frequently to several sources:

ES   E. Smith, *The Compleat Housewife: or Accomplish'd Gentlewoman's Companion* (1753)

JG   John Gerard, *Herball* (1597)

JW   John Wesley, *Primitive Remedies* (1776)

LIA   *Ladies' Indispensable Assistant* (1852)

MB   Mrs. Beeton, *Book of Household Management* (1861)

NC   Nicholas Culpeper, *English Physician and Complete Herbal* (1652)

OFA   *The Old Farmer's Almanac*

Chapter 1

Kitchen Gardens & Medicinal Herbs

Yarrow
(Achillea millefolium)

*Show me your garden and I
shall tell you what you are.*

— ALFRED AUSTIN (1835–1913)

A Kitchen-Garden don't thrive better or faster in any part of the Universe than there," said Robert Beverly, in 1705, in a book intended to lure prospective settlers to Virginia. He was speaking of the "potherbs," medicinal herbs, small fruits, and berries that were commonly grown in the protected dooryards of early American households. The potherb was any plant whose leaves, stems, roots, or flowers were cooked and eaten or used as a seasoning. The picture Beverly painted of these early kitchen gardens — private, sunny enclosures of bountiful production — might be our first step toward more healthful eating.

Kitchen gardens are best explained through the etymology of the word "garden," which evolves through various branches of "yard" — *geard, garthy, garda,* a sheltered or protected place for some special purpose. They were handy and generally south-facing. A simple fence or box hedge kept out the cows and hens, and the plants were chosen primarily for their culinary and medicinal usefulness. Sometimes called a woman's garden or a cottage garden, kitchen gardens were distinguished from the orchard or "falling garden," from the "pleasure garden" of purely ornamental flowers, or from the more distant fields. Later, in the early 1800s, some of these were refined into the "parlor garden," with more formal designs for the paths and beds and more ornamental plantings. In the earlier kitchen gardens, however, form definitely followed function.

A Garden of Useful Plants

The plant selections for kitchen gardens were, above all, useful. They could include medicinals, flavorings, small and frequently used vegetables, herbal insect repellents and room deodorants, or plants for dyeing or teasing wool or flax. Any tender plants that needed the added warmth from a stone foundation or protection from wind and weather would be candidates for the kitchen garden. A midwife's garden might be more heavily laden with medicinals, while a spinner and weaver's garden would favor dyeplants and teasels. Purely ornamental flowers were not apt to be found here (unless they had been brought from England for sentimental reasons), but many plants were in bloom. The lavenders, flowering thyme, yarrow, bee balm, and lupines were among the medicinals, after all.

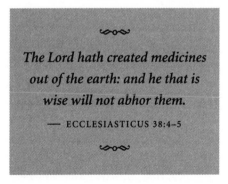

The Lord hath created medicines out of the earth: and he that is wise will not abhor them.

— ECCLESIASTICUS 38:4–5

Immediately outside the kitchen dooryard were the most common potherbs brought to America by the colonists, or, as John Lawrence, in *The Clergyman's Recreation* (1726), labeled them, "some of those Reptiles useful in the Kitchen, viz Carrots, Onions, Parsnips, Spinage, etc." Some of these "Reptiles," like spinach, were prepared in virtually the same ways they are today — boiled or steamed, possibly served with bacon or hard-cooked egg, and flavored with butter or pepper. Others that we would not generally cook today, such as various lettuces, were also boiled or wilted before serving and were generally well spiced and dripping with butter or salad dressing.

Native edibles were frequently added to the kitchen fare but probably gathered somewhat farther afield, including dandelions, cowslip greens, rhubarb, sarsaparilla, cresses, asparagus, and horseradish. Hops were another native edible which could be gathered wild, but they were often given room in the kitchen garden for expediency. They were used in bread making, salads, to flavor beer, in preserving, and for medicinal purposes.

Besides the handiness of a kitchen garden for harvesting purposes, there was the convenience of having its upkeep close at hand and under one's watchful eye. Translated to the modern day, the colonial kitchen garden has several virtues to recommend it. No one would argue with the aesthetic beauty of a flower garden, nor the aromatic herb garden, and clearly those qualities remain desirable today. Companion gardening techniques still argue that we do well to mix our vegetables and herbs, for better yields and soil improvement, just as they were combined and rotated in the colonial kitchen gardens. And

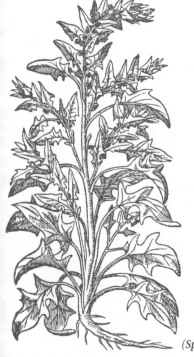

Spinach
(Spinacia oleracea)

anyone who has opted for a row of lettuce close to the kitchen knows that you eat more salads that way. Perhaps above all is the ever-present invitation to come outdoors that a kitchen garden seems to inspire.

We are less apt to garden for medicinals today, although many of us continue to depend on lavender to scent our closets and aloe to treat burns. Hen-and-chickens, or houseleek, is also a handy salve for stings and minor burns and looks ornamental besides. A strong sage tea soothes sunburns, and a bit of sage burned in a fireplace or chafing dish makes a great room freshener. Many of the common mints and other herbs make relaxing, natural teas to sip for the ease of today's stresses. These and other herbal remedies are available to anyone who chooses to learn them. A kitchen garden offers both an attractive space for these plants and the daily reminder to study and make use of what we sow.

Houseleek
(*Sempervivum soboliferum*)

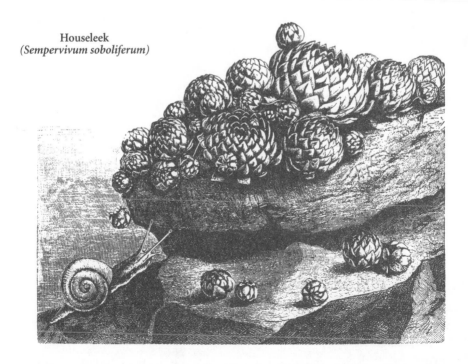

Identifying & Harvesting Plants

For most of us, it's best to purchase the remedy ingredients we need from a reliable source, such as a trusted health food store or pharmacy. Gardeners may want to experiment with growing their own ingredients and can do so with ease and safety as long as they double-check the Latin names when obtaining seeds or starter plants. Also, some seeds, such as celery, are frequently sold horticulturally with fungicides applied to them and should not be used for medicinals. Similarly, stick with organic fertilizers in your "physic garden."

Harvesting in the wild is best left to the experts. Although most of us can safely identify the common burdock or dandelion, less distinctive plants are remarkably similar in appearance to other more toxic plants, and the confusion could make you sick. For example, angelica is easily confused with water hemlock. Sweet cicely, parsley, and fennel can be easily mistaken for poison hemlock. Besides physical similarities between plants, some distinct plants share a common name or have very similar sounding names (such as barberry, bearberry, and bayberry). Again, the Latin names are your best guide.

If you feel confident enough to risk harvesting your own plants, be on the lookout for possible contaminants in the soil or air where they thrive. Have those dandelions on the lawn survived a treatment of weed killer? If so, don't eat them. Is the burdock growing next to a multi-lane highway where automobiles are polluting the environment? Maybe it won't be so cleansing to your system.

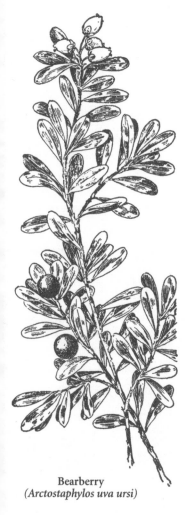

Bearberry
(*Arctostaphylos uva ursi*)

Collecting Herbs

Most herbs are harvested for their leaves, so the trick is to gather them when they are chock full of the essential oils that give them their flavor and fragrance. According to herbalist Nicholas Culpeper's *English Physician and Complete Herbal* (1652), "The leaves of such herbs as run up to seed are not so good when they are in flower as before." Another early guide recommends gathering the herbs when the flower has budded but not yet opened. Obviously, if you want the flower or seed, you'll have to wait longer for your harvest.

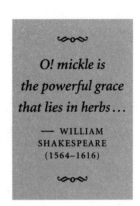

O! mickle is the powerful grace that lies in herbs...

— WILLIAM SHAKESPEARE (1564–1616)

As a general guide, take roots in the fall (folklore claims that roots taken in their growing season will shrink to nothing), bark in the late winter or early spring, leaves and herb stems when the plant is just short of bloom, flowers when they first open, and seeds when first ripe. Dry the plant parts slowly in the shade and make sure they're thoroughly dry so they won't mold (unless you want a fermented tea, or oolong).

Many gardeners recommend lightly watering the herbs the evening before your harvest so that the plants are clean and can dry on the stem. Then wait until after the morning dew has dried, but before the sun is hot enough to volatilize oils, to harvest. Annuals should be completely harvested, perennials pruned by about a third. In the case of perennials, be sure you allow time for vigorous regrowth before winter to avoid winterkilled plants.

Hang the herbs in small bunches or strip the leaves and lay them on clean paper or screens. Put them outdoors in the shade during the day (you'll have to bring them in at night to avoid dampness or dew) or in a dry attic or shed. Drying is the same for flowers and seeds. Once the plant parts are brittle and dry, bottle them to retain their flavor.

Chapter 2

Infusions, Decoctions & Tinctures

Roman Chamomile
(Chamaemelum nobile)

Now stir the fire, and close the shutters fast,
Let fall the curtains, wheel the sofa round,
And while the bubbling and loud-hissing urn
Throws up a steamy column, and the cups
That cheer but not inebriate wait on each,
So let us welcome peaceful evening in.

— *WILLIAM COWPER (1731–1800)*

olklore suggests that a singing teakettle brings pleasant news. We're also warned never to let the kettle go dry, or bad luck will follow. Over the centuries, we've come to recognize that chamomile tea is calming, red clover tea is good for sore throats, raspberry and blackberry leaves are good for blending, and rose hip tea is full of vitamin C. We may not be aware that bergamot (helpful for coughs and fevers) gives Earl Grey its characteristic flavor, but we enjoy it anyway. Perhaps it's no coincidence that both the discovery of tea and the origins of medical knowledge have been attributed to the same person, the Chinese "Yellow Emperor" (c. 2500 B.C.), who may have saved his people from a cholera epidemic by insisting that they boil their water. Since tea leaves were often added to the water, various teas became associated with curative powers. In Japan, the meditative aspect of the tea ceremony assumed restorative properties. Can a simple cup of tea and other herbal remedies be the key to health?

Mrs. Beeton, in her *Book of Household Management* (1861), listed tea as "the cup that cheers but not inebriates," quoting William Cowper. At about the same time, Florence Nightingale remarked on how tea had acquired an almost mystical place in English sickrooms: "A great deal too much against tea is said by wise people, and a great deal too much of tea is given to the sick by foolish people." Her point was that tea, while certainly restorative, could not replace more nutritious fare. Let's look at teas, then, as a starting point, a beginning of the many small steps that can be taken toward learning and using herbal remedies.

Depending on the ingredients used, tea can be a preventive medicine, a restorative, or simply a thirst-quenching and relaxing treat. The tannic acid in tea has been prescribed to counteract alkaline toxins, which include morphine and other opiates, nicotine, strychnine, and caffeine. Some teas are used to reduce blood cholesterol, as stimulants, or as astringents. Green teas have been recommended as diuretics and to counteract tumors. Whatever else they may do, it's reasonably safe to assume that most teas "never do harm to anyone," as Hippocrates, the Greek "Father of Medicine," would have wished. (Strictly speaking, he did not write the Hippocratic oath but merely espoused it.) Consider the cup of tea as a vehicle for transmitting the healing powers of a whole range of different herbs, but choose those herbs carefully. Some, such as comfrey, can do harm (see Appendix I).

An individual should always bow before the curative powers of the chamomile plant.
— SLOVAKIAN SAYING

Infusions & Tisanes

An infusion is one form of tea making. Make yourself a cup of tea. Let it steep a little longer, maybe 10 to 20 minutes, and that's an infusion. Some call it a tisane. The soluble elements of, say, peppermint (or whatever your choice of herbs) are unlocked into the hot water and made available to you by your inhaling the steam, drinking the liquid, or perhaps applying it externally as an antiseptic wash. Not all infusions are meant to be sipped; some are intended as rinses, for use via compresses, as foot soaks, to massage into the skin, or for use aromatically. An infusion may have a single ingredient or many. It may be ingested hot or cold, inhaled as a vapor, used to perfume a pillow to relieve stress or insomnia, or enjoyed in your bath.

Decoctions, or When to Boil

If your medicinal plant is tougher — say, the bark, roots, rhizomes, seeds, nuts, or woody stems — then you need a more intensive tea-making process. Bring the ingredient to a boil in water, cover, and let simmer for 10 to 20 minutes. That's a decoction, from the Latin *de* (down) and *coquere* (to cook). Boiling or simmering is required to extract the concentrated elements you seek. Lemon balm and horehound generally require boiling. Some herbalists suggest that you should soak the bark or plant parts overnight in cool water, then bring them to a boil. Like infusions, decoctions may contain one ingredient or many, may be ingested hot or cold, or may be otherwise applied.

Tough wintergreen leaves, broken and simmered in water, can be decocted to make a cooling, external pain reliever for bruises and swelling. Mint leaves or chamomile flowers, however, either fresh or dried, are more fragile and require just a light infusion. Decocting will evaporate their fragrant oils. Both infusions and decoctions can be refrigerated and then reheated a day or two later. Or they may be converted into syrups by heating them with sugar or honey, making them more palatable for children.

Tinctures, or Chemical Extractions

A tincture is another method of extracting the beneficial substance from a plant, this time by soaking it for some time in a solvent such as alcohol. The process may take several weeks or more. Resins and gums require up to 90 percent alcohol to extract the essential substance, while a glycoside (such as soapwort, mullein, dock, or licorice) or a tannin (such as witch hazel) might require only 25 percent. Brandy, gin, and vodka have all been used with good results. Alcohol-based tinctures tend to be highly concentrated, and the dosage is given in drops or teaspoons. (Take care to use proper doses.) Alcohol also acts as a preservative, so tinctures can be kept, unrefrigerated, for two years and sometimes longer.

Vinegars (generally apple cider vinegar) and glycerol (glycerin) have been used to extract alkaloids, minerals, and vitamins, but they don't have the extracting

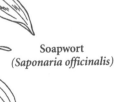

Soapwort
(*Saponaria officinalis*)

*Thank God for tea!
What would
the world do
without tea? —
how did it exist?
I am glad I was not
born before tea.*

— SYDNEY SMITH
(1769–1845)

power of alcohol. Herbal vinegars, such as the tarragon vinegar now common in markets, are basically vinegar-based tinctures of very mild potency. Glycerol is sweeter than either alcohol or vinegar and consequently is often used for children's remedies or for someone who can't tolerate alcohol.

Tinctures are commonly made with a single ingredient, although they may be combined in various ways to form a remedy. Very bitter herbs are often made into tinctures and then combined with sweetened teas or otherwise camouflaged. Health food stores and herb shops usually carry an assortment of commercially made tinctures, some of which (such as goldenseal and purple coneflower [echinacea]) may come ready-mixed in remedy form. If you make your own tinctures for long-term use, you should strain the bottled liquid through cheesecloth to remove the plant solids and keep the tincture from spoiling. Some avid gardeners purchase a small wine press or a hydraulic jack to press their extracted herbs for higher yield and potency. (**Caution!** Do not try to dilute a tincture or an essential oil with water and use it as you would an infusion or a decoction. You're likely to get too high a dose.)

Purple coneflower
(*Echinacea purpurea*)

Remedies for Respiratory Troubles

Following are various old remedies for the "unknown guests" (ailments) that visit in the respiratory system — that is, in the nose, throat, larynx, trachea, bronchi, and lungs. We've also listed fevers here, since they're often (but not always) a result of respiratory infections. Earaches are treated in this section as well.

Do not be fooled into thinking that the simplest remedies are the least beneficial. Modern science has recently thrown its weight behind the former "old wives' tales" of hot chicken soup and almost anything containing garlic as effective treatments for cold symptoms. Indeed, some studies suggest that virtually any inhaled steam is beneficial, so a cup of steaming herbal tea should not be dismissed as lacking preventive and restorative powers. Likewise, do not dismiss persistent respiratory ailments as being too minor for expert diagnosis and advice.

COLDS

❦ Make a sandwich of whole-wheat bread, raw yellow onion, a good half inch of horseradish, Cheddar cheese, and brown mustard. A daily dose will prevent the common cold.

❦ Feed a cold, starve a fever.

❦ Take chicken soup steaming hot and seasoned with garlic.

❦ Ingest raw garlic to stop a sneezing fit. Also, eat a few cloves of garlic to fight an infection, then chew parsley for the breath. Take fennel or ginger tea if the garlic upsets your stomach.

❦ Use garlic, onions, thyme, sage, and vitamin C regularly to help prevent colds and infections.

❦ Let dishes drip-dry; don't wipe them with a towel, which spreads germs. Wash your hands often. Don't share towels or bathroom cups. Turn the heat down to 68° F or below and humidify the air in winter months. If you humidify with a stovetop pan of water, add cinnamon and cloves to the water and change it regularly.

❦ Hot Buttered Rum: Put 1 teaspoon brown sugar in a mug, sprinkle in some ground cloves and a dab of butter, add a jigger of rum, and fill with boiling water. Stir with a cinnamon stick. Good for colds and chills.

❦ Drink hot water laced with lemon juice and honey.

Thyme
(Thymus vulgaris)

SORE THROATS

❧ Drink any hot liquid.

❧ Suck on horehound drops.

❧ Suck on zinc lozenges.

❧ Add salt and pepper to apple cider vinegar and gargle with the mixture.

❧ Gargle frequently with warm salt water.

❧ Make a syrup of horseradish, lemon juice, and honey to relieve a sore throat and treat laryngitis. (**Caution!** This can be hard on the stomach.)

❧ In Germany, a cool sage tea gargle is used for sore throats.

❧ Take a decoction of elecampane roots.

❧ Make a decoction of turnips, sweeten with honey or sugar, and drink before bedtime. Good for coughs and hoarseness.

❧ Gargle with a warm infusion of agrimony, sage, or rosemary or with a tincture of purple coneflower.

❧ "Apply a chin stay (a band under the chin) of roasted figs. Or, snuff a little honey up your nose. Or, live on apples and apple water. Or, for the putrid sore throat, take a lump of sugar in brandy." (JW)

❧ "For hoarseness, apply garlic to the feet, apply a mustard plaster to the chest, ingest a conserve of roses, eat powdered nettle roots in molasses, or take boiled wheat bran with water and honey." (JW)

Slippery elm (*Ulmus rubra*)

Slippery Elm Jelly

slippery elm flour*
sugar
teacup of cold water

nutmeg or other spice
pint of cold water

Mix together a large spoonful each of slippery elm flour and sugar. Stir into the teacup of water and season with nutmeg or any agreeable spice. Pour into the pint of water. Boil, and it is finished. The jelly may be made thick or thin and seasoned to suit your taste.

From an unpublished recipe book, c. 1850.

*Available from most health food stores and some pharmacies.

ASTHMA

❦ Drink chamomile tea, a natural antihistamine. Or, decoct Roman chamomile flowers and inhale the steam.

❦ If your asthma is allergy based and pollen is the source of your trouble, add honey to any tea and drink it in frequent doses to build up your immunity. Or, dilute honey with an equal amount of water or lemon juice and take by the tablespoon as a remedial syrup. ("The hand that gave the wound must give the cure.")

❦ Grate some horseradish and sniff of it liberally to clear the sinuses and stimulate easier breathing.

❦ Suck horehound candy or make a tea of decocted horehound leaves.

❦ Inhale eucalyptus in a bouquet, from a scented pillow or sachet, or from a heat ring treated with a couple of drops of the essential oil.

❦ Make a tea of equal parts decocted vervain (verbena), horehound, and elecampane roots. Simmer for about 20 minutes, strain, and cool. Drink about 1 pint three times a day.

❦ "Drink a decoction of apples (boiling water poured over sliced apples). Or, keep your feet warm, promote perspiration, and exercise. Or, drink mullein or sweet marjoram tea." (JW)

❦ Drink a tea made of horehound, hyssop, sage, or yarrow. Or, sip a potion made by steeping 4 quarts huckleberries for 4 days in 2 gallons good gin.

❦ "Take the root of skunk cabbage, and boil it until very strong, then strain off the liquor; to which add, one table-spoon of garlic juice to one pint of the liquor, and simmer them together. Dose, one table-spoonful, three times a day." (LIA)

❦ "Take a table-spoonful of English or white mustard seed, in molasses or water, morning and evening." (LIA)

Asthma Alleviator

1 pint Irish moss jelly*
½ yellow onion
2 cloves garlic
½ cup honey

Combine the Irish moss jelly, onion, and garlic in a saucepan and simmer for 30 minutes. Strain through a sieve and add the honey. Take 1 tablespoon every couple of hours as needed.

*Irish moss is a North Atlantic seaweed. The jelly is available at health food stores and some pharmacies.

Irish moss
(*Chondrus crispus*)

COUGHS

❦ Take a phlegm-reducing infusion made with hyssop, anise, elder, or goldenrod.

❦ Make a tea of horehound, ground ivy, angelica, red clover, wild cherry, or elecampane roots. Add lemon and honey if desired.

❦ Drink an infusion of honeysuckle leaves and flowers.

❦ "Cough Elecampane: Make a syrup by slicing the fresh root[s], covering them with sugar, and baking them for an hour or two." (LIA)

❦ Decoct quince seeds, about 1 ounce to 1 cup boiling water. Let sit for 1 hour, strain, and take with an equal amount of honey as a cough syrup or for hoarseness or a sore throat.

❦ Make a pectoral (chest plaster, see Chapter 3) of sage, barley, and turnips.

❦ Make a chest poultice of boiled onions.

❦ Make a mustard plaster with egg whites and flaxseed meal, applied over a piece of gauze. Check at regular intervals to avoid burning or irritating the skin.

❦ Native Americans decocted pine pitch or dried balsamroot to make a strong tea.

❦ Induce sweating.

❦ Take a hot bath with eucalyptus in the water. (**Caution!** Check first to be sure it doesn't irritate your skin. And never take eucalyptus oil internally; it's highly poisonous.)

❦ Drink mullein flower tea.

❦ Treat the "pneumony fever" with a tea of onions and wild lobelia. (**Caution!** If it's a cough, you might try this. If it's pneumonia, see your doctor.)

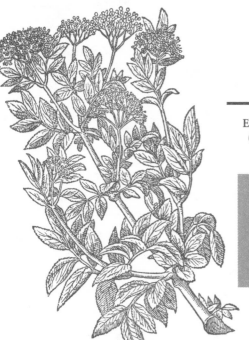

Elder
(*Sambucus nigra*)

∽○∾

Love, and a cough, cannot be hid.

— GEORGE HERBERT (1593–1632)

∽○∾

Horehound Lozenges

1 cup horehound leaves
1 cup water
2 cups sugar
2 tablespoons corn syrup or honey

Boil the horehound leaves in the water for 20 minutes. Cool well. Strain the mixture through cheesecloth, reserving the decocted liquid and discarding the dregs (good compost). Add the sugar and corn syrup or honey to the liquid. Boil again, then reduce the heat to a simmer. Cook, stirring constantly, until the syrup reaches the hard-crack stage (300° F).

Butter a baking sheet and pour in the syrup. When the candy has cooled slightly, score and break into drop-size pieces. Roll in granulated sugar if desired. Use as cough lozenges (an expectorant). (**Caution!** In large doses, horehound acts as a purgative and may precipitate an irregular heartbeat.)

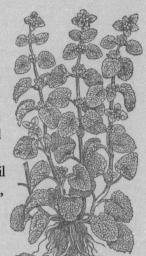

Black horehound
(Ballota nigra)

CATARRH

Catarrh is generally defined as the overproduction of mucus, often resulting from an infection or inflammation.

❦ Make a tea of boneset, peppermint, elder flowers, and yarrow to help break up the mucus congestion and reduce fever.

❦ Decoct ginger, cinnamon stick, cloves, and coriander seed. Make it into a tea and sweeten with honey.

❦ Eat raw garlic.

❦ Make a footbath with powdered mustard.

❦ Add cayenne pepper to your cooking to break up congestion.

❦ Inhale the steam of chamomile tea.

❦ Make a tea or syrup of decocted elecampane.

FEVER

High body temperatures or alternating chills and fever are the body's way of responding to an infection. A very high fever (102° F and up) or a prolonged fever indicates the need for professional advice. Children's fevers often require professional care, since they may result from streptococcal or other bacterial infections that can be dangerous if not properly treated. For nonbacterial fevers, remedies are either cooling, such as boneset or peppermint (to encourage sweating), or warming, such as cayenne pepper or ginger (to maintain body heat).

🐾 Drink chamomile tea or warm lemonade to reduce a fever.

🐾 "A Drink for a Fever: Take a quart of spring water, an ounce of burnt hartshorn, a nutmeg quarter'd, and a stick of cinnamon; let it boil a quarter of an hour; when it is cold sweeten it to your taste with syrup of lemons, or fine sugar, with as many drops of spirit of vitriol as will just sharpen it. Drink of this when you please." (ES)

🐾 Native Americans took boneset tea, once used for "breakbone fever" (an acute, infectious tropical disease). This can upset the stomach.

🐾 Make a tea of yarrow, angelica, mulberry leaves, barberry berries, elder flowers, ground ivy, peppermint, catnip, or vervain (verbena). Catnip helps reduce mucus.

🐾 For chills, take fresh gingerroot.

🐾 Take cayenne pepper (in food, broth, or tea) to warm the body, promote sweating, and enhance the body's infection-fighting ability.

🐾 "To avoid fall fevers, eat moderately, drink sparingly, lie not down on the damp earth, nor overheat yourself; but keep your temper, and change your clothes as the weather changes." (OFA, 1852)

🐾 "Fever and Ague: Take of cloves and cream of tartar, each half an ounce, and one ounce of Peruvian bark, mix in a little tea, molasses or honey, and take it on the well days in such quantities as the stomach will bear." (LIA)

So, when a raging fever burns,
We shift from side to side by turns;
And 't is a poor relief we gain
To change the place, but keep the pain.

— ISAAC WATTS (1674–1748)

EARACHE

Never drop anything into the ear if there is evidence (such as fluid or a waxy discharge emanating from the ear) that the eardrum has been punctured. In this case, consult your health practitioner, perhaps using dry heat in the meantime.

❦ Many earaches are offshoots of colds, flu, or other congestion. If this is the case, reduce the mucus and phlegm with a tea of goldenseal, purple coneflower, eyebright, or elder flowers.

❦ In mild cases or while you're waiting for a medical treatment to take effect, try using a hair dryer, on its coolest setting and held a good six inches away, to blow warm air into a child's ear. Both the white noise of the dryer and the dry heat will help ease the symptoms and calm a fussy child.

❦ A warm heating pad on the pillow can ease mild earaches.

❦ Many of the older generation recall their parents boiling an onion and placing pieces of the warm onion on the affected ear. Some used warmed "sweet oil" (olive oil) as eardrops.

❦ Make an infusion or tincture of mullein and use it cold as eardrops.

❦ Use oil of fennel or bruised fennel seeds, applied externally, to ease an earache.

❦ "Take a table-spoon of fine salt, and tie it up in a little bag, heat it quite hot, and lay it on the ear, shifting it several times; and it will afford speedy relief." (LIA)

❦ Combine equal parts white vinegar and rubbing alcohol and put one or two drops in each ear three times a day as an antiseptic to prevent ear infections or so-called swimmer's ear.

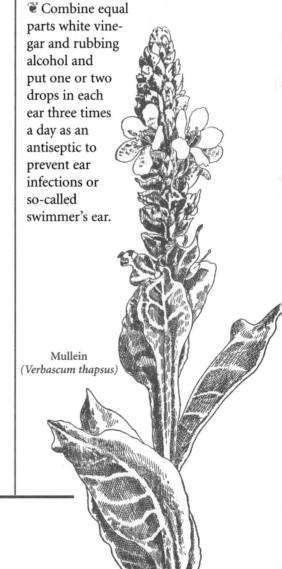

Mullein
(*Verbascum thapsus*)

Chapter 3

Poultices, Salves & Ointments

To use on . . . wounds and broken arms
Some had their salves and others worked their charms,
And sage they drank, and likewise remedies
Of herbs, for they would save their limbs with these.

— GEOFFREY CHAUCER (C. 1340–1400)

Sage
(Salvia officinalis)

Some early salves and poultices were unsavory concoctions of ingredients such as urine, manure, "flayed Mouse," mashed earthworms, dried fox lungs, eel gall, hare brains, and crab eyes, as any reading of the 17th-century herbalist Nicholas Culpeper will tell you. One early American belief was that pouring vinegar on the hinge of a door after you saw a shooting star would make your warts go away. Other superstitions advised carrying a buckeye (horse chestnut) in your pocket to prevent rheumatism. Copper bracelets, gold rings, red strings, and a nail from a horseshoe were reputed to "stay arthritis." And whatever the news of your family, good or bad, you must tell it to the bees and seek their blessing; otherwise, they might swarm and deprive you of their honey, a critical ingredient in countless remedies.

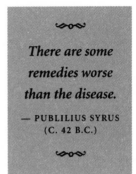

> *There are some remedies worse than the disease.*
>
> — PUBLILIUS SYRUS
> (C. 42 B.C.)

Both Culpeper's *English Physician and Complete Herbal* (1652) and "W.M." of *The Queen's Closet Opened* (1656) agreed on sage for the teeth and mouth. Whether in a hot infusion or a gargle, a leaf for rubbing the teeth after meals, or a dried stem to use as a toothpick, sage was the dental herb. "If you will keep your teeth from rotting, or aching, wash the mouth continually every morning with juyce of Lemons, and afterward rub your teeth with a Sage-leaf, or else with a little Nutmeg in powder; also wash your mouth with a little fair water after meats," Culpeper advised. For a toothache, colonial American superstitions included packing the hollow with gunpowder or ground cloves. If that didn't work, you could try chewing garlic, tobacco, or hops. A spider enclosed in a nutshell was prescribed as a helpful amulet. Still desperate? John Wesley (*Primitive Remedies*, 1776) tried being electrified through the teeth, which he recommended. Personally, we prefer prevention.

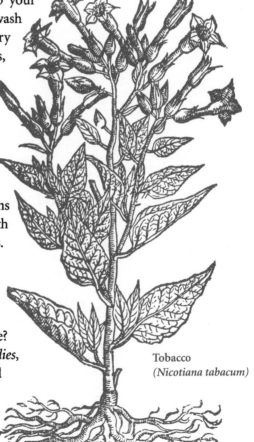

Tobacco
(*Nicotiana tabacum*)

Poultices, Plasters & Compresses

Simply speaking, a poultice or plaster is a mixture of dried or fresh herbs, dampened with water or oil, and applied externally to the chest or some other area to stimulate the affected part. Generally, a poultice implies a hot application, whereas a plaster might be applied at room temperature. According to *The American Heritage Dictionary* (3rd ed.), *poultice* derives its meaning from the Latin word for "paste." It also may come from the Greek word for "porridge," because bread or meal, as well as clay or some other adhesive substance, was often used to make the herb mixture into a damp paste. Native Americans frequently used the pitch from pine, spruce, or hemlock trees to make a salve to bind broken bones. The pitch would harden into a "strengthening plaster" and help keep the bone in place during healing. Chewing a leaf of plantain and spitting the bits onto a bug bite is a crude form of poultice making. Sometimes a poultice might consist of a single, broad leaf, such as a cabbage or tobacco leaf, bound with a damp cloth and kept moist with the heat of a hot-water bottle or heating pad. Because mustard and other such ingredients can be irritating to the skin, many poultices are best applied between layers of gauze so that they can be easily lifted, checked for results, and neatly removed when appropriate.

A compress, also called a fomentation, is simpler still, made of a clean cloth (terry cloth, flannel, cheesecloth, gauze, and chamois are often used) dipped in a liquid. A warm compress might be made with a

Plantain
(*Plantago major*)

washcloth soaked in a chamomile or dill infusion and applied to the forehead to relieve a stress headache, insomnia, or tired eyes. An inflamed, arthritic elbow would typically be wrapped in a hot compress.

Salves, Ointments & Liniments

Salves and ointments are essentially creams or lotions in a variety of formulas. Most start with an herb or herb blend macerated in oil, such as olive oil or almond oil (often combined in equal parts), then mixed with warmed beeswax, petroleum jelly, or a water-based cream. If petroleum jelly is used, the herbs are generally macerated in mineral oil.

Liniments are simply oil-based formulas, made *without* waxes, creams, or jellies. Liniments, such as "baby oil" or aromatic almond oil, are generally massaged into the skin. A liniment may contain a heat-producing ingredient, such as cayenne pepper, horseradish, ginger, or mustard, to increase circulation and act as a counterirritant for muscle swelling. The idea is to increase the blood flow to that area so that it is cleansed through a more stimulating circulation. You may hear liniments called embrocations or rube-facients. A weak solution of powdered mustard in oil (or even hot water) is a rudimentary, surprisingly effective form of a liniment for arthritis or rheumatic disorders.

Black Mustard
(Brassica nigra)

Fragrant Herb Oil and Antibacterial Salve

This oil can be used as a pleasantly fragrant massage agent for sore muscles, combined with boiling water and inhaled for nasal congestion, or combined with softened beeswax to make an antibacterial salve for skin problems.

> **equal parts almond oil and olive oil**
> **fresh peppermint leaves (or other aromatic herb), enough to loosely fill jar**
> **1 tablespoon rubbing alcohol, to discourage mold**
> **a few drops benzoin tincture, to keep herb oil stable (available at pharmacies and health food stores)**

Put the peppermint leaves in a glass jar and cover with the oil mixture. Add the rubbing alcohol. Cover the jar, put on a sunny windowsill, and let this solar infusion steep for at least 2 weeks. Strain and bottle the infused oil. (The strained dregs make good compost.) Add the benzoin tincture.

To make the antibacterial salve, heat equal parts beeswax and herb oil — enough to fill a small lip balm container. Some herbalists like to add equal parts vitamin E oil (good for any skin treatment) and anhydrous lanolin (also available at pharmacies and health food stores) along with the beeswax and herb oil. The more beeswax you add, the firmer the salve.

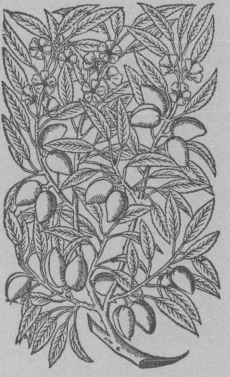

Almond (*Amygdalus communis*)

RHEUMATISM & ARTHRITIS

Rheumatism is a generic term that encompasses swelling, soreness, stiffness, and aching of the joints, including arthritis, bursitis, and rheumatic fever. A plant called rheumatism root or wild yam is commonly prescribed in domestic remedy books.

❦ Take 10 to 30 drops of a tincture of rheumatism root in water up to three times a day.

❦ Combine tinctures of rheumatism root, burdock root, motherwort, and black cohosh (roughly equal parts rheumatism root and burdock root, one-half part motherwort, and one-quarter part black cohosh). Take in water as needed.

❦ Make a salve of cayenne pepper and apply externally to inflamed joints as a counterirritant to add soothing heat to the aching area.

❦ Native Americans made a poultice of sage, tobacco, angelica, balsam, or the tops of the creosote bush for rheumatism.

❦ Drink cilantro (coriander) tea, made from the dried leaves and/or seeds. The plant form is cilantro, also called Chinese parsley. The seeds are coriander, frequently used in Indian recipes.

❦ Drink a tea made of celery seed, purple coneflower, and burdock to build up your resistance.

❦ Use turmeric in your food. Or, take a drink of warm milk with 1 teaspoon ground turmeric up to three times a day to reduce the swelling of arthritis.

❦ Make an infusion of dried meadowsweet and sip it as a tea. (**Caution!** Meadowsweet contains salicin, the healing ingredient in aspirin, so heed the same precautions as for aspirin. Pregnant women and children at risk of Reye's syndrome should avoid it.)

❦ Take a teaspoon of crushed garlic twice a day with a liquid.

❦ "Make a plaster of poplar bark by taking the bark of the root, boiling it down in water to an extract, mixing it with a little spirit, and applying it to the rheumatism or any other pain." (LIA)

Meadowsweet
(*Spiraea latifolia*)

❧ "Recipe for Rheumatism: Take 4 ounces Castile soap; 2 ounces Camphor; half an ounce Oil Rosemary; 3 pints Alcohol. Soak the soap three days in the Alcohol and then add the other ingredients. Apply externally." (LIA)

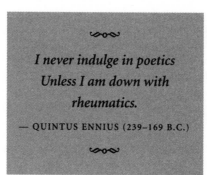

I never indulge in poetics Unless I am down with rheumatics.

— QUINTUS ENNIUS (239–169 B.C.)

❧ Drink a tea made of decocted pussy willow or slippery elm bark.

❧ Induce sweating.

❧ For extreme cases, honeybee stings on the affected area have been reputed to give relief.

❧ If you are overweight, lose weight so that your joints will have fewer pounds to carry. Even a small weight loss can make a difference.

❧ For creaky joints in hands or other accessible areas, "bathe" the area under the heat of a light bulb in a desk lamp (12 inches away). For less accessible areas, try a heating pad.

❧ For bursitis, make a poultice of decocted comfrey or cabbage leaves, mashed and applied warm between layers of gauze. Other soothing herbs include marshmallow, linseed (crushed flaxseed), and slippery elm. (**Caution!** Do not take comfrey internally.)

❧ Boil hot apple cider vinegar with cayenne pepper, cool somewhat, and apply to bursitis via a compress. Check frequently to make sure the cayenne doesn't irritate the skin. It should bring heat but not burn.

❧ Wash the affected parts in a hot-water bath with powdered mustard (in a weak solution).

❧ Some arthritis sufferers note the homeopathic use of arnica as having helped them dramatically.

❧ Ginkgo is sometimes advertised as being beneficial for arthritis and rheumatism.

INSECT BITES & STINGS

If you are stung and the insect has left its stinger in you, try to remove it by scraping the skin lightly or pressing it sideways with a fingernail or tweezers. Allergic reactions to bee stings can cause dangerous swelling of air passages and require emergency medical attention. If you have any symptoms of an allergic reaction, get immediate help from a doctor.

🌿 Crush the flower of red clover and apply to insect bites and stings.

🌿 Apply a poultice of bee balm for bee stings. The same thing will ward off mosquitoes.

🌿 "Combine equal parts baking soda and salt in warm water and rub in to relieve the itching and pain caused by insect bites or stings." (OFA, 1917)

🌿 "Apply mud to bee or wasp stings." (OFA, 1943)

🌿 Chew plantain leaves and apply the macerated leaves to the bite as a poultice.

🌿 Rub a slice of cucumber on an ant bite.

🌿 Apply jewelweed juice. Or, make jewelweed ice cubes: Fill a pot with jewelweed stems and leaves and cover with water. Reduce by one-half and freeze in ice cube trays. (**Caution!** Label well.) Use externally to cool and soothe bites and stings. You can keep the cubes indefinitely.

🌿 Dilute lavender oil or cinnamon oil and apply to bites and stings.

🌿 Decoct natural antiseptics such as garlic, dogwood, oak bark, sphagnum moss, or witch hazel and use as a wash for bites and stings.

🌿 Garlic "fights dangerous infirmities and makes snakes, serpents, and other small beasts hide. Together with honey it is useful against dog bites; mixed with oil it heals poisoned wounds and ulcerations." (16TH-CENTURY HERBAL)

🌿 Apply onion juice, garlic juice, or radish juice.

🌿 Apply vinegar, lemon juice, or a vinaigrette-type salad dressing.

🌿 Apply the juice from a mullein leaf or a tobacco leaf.

🌿 Apply a paste of ground cloves and water.

🌿 For the sting of stinging nettles, apply the juice from the stems of the same plant.

Horseradish Tincture

½ cup grated horseradish root
1 pint rubbing alcohol

Submerge the horseradish in the alcohol for 2 to 3 days. Shake the mixture a couple of times a day. Strain off the grated root. Bottle the liquid and cap tightly. The resulting tincture is useful for bug bites and stings, minor skin wounds, and superficial infections.

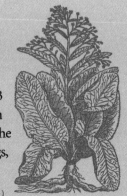

Horseradish (*Armoracia rusticana*)

POISON IVY & OTHER ITCHING

Never try to burn poison ivy to remove it from the premises; inhaling the smoke can cause severe and dangerous reactions. Anytime the throat, eyes, face, or genitalia are involved in a case of poison ivy, oak, or sumac, consult your doctor. Sensitive individuals can contract poison ivy indirectly, such as by petting cats and dogs that may have been in contact with the plants. If the juice of the plants has been smeared on clothing or garden tools, it can remain active for up to a year. Simple washing will remove it. Likewise, once exposed areas of the skin have been washed, the poison ivy will no longer be spread by skin-to-skin contact or by oozing from the rash.

❦ To rid yourself of poison ivy juice after you are first exposed, wash well with soap and water, then give yourself a sponge bath with rubbing alcohol to thoroughly remove it. If any rash, blisters, and sores have developed, omit the rubbing alcohol and just wash well. Wash clothes, tools, and pets that may have been contaminated as well.

❦ Crush jewelweed stems and the swollen nodes — not the roots — and apply the juice to a poison ivy or poison oak rash. Some people say that jewelweed juice can be applied as a preventive if you think you may encounter poison ivy. Jewelweed often grows near poison ivy, in shady spots of deep, moist woods.

❦ Stinging nettles also may grow near poison ivy. Use nettle juice from the stems to treat unintentional contact with either one. This is also good for eczema.

❦ Native Americans used mugwort juice to treat poison ivy.

❦ Chew plantain and apply directly as a poultice to poison ivy or other itchy rashes. Or, make an infusion or salve from fresh or dried plantain leaves. Or, gather plantain seeds from the seed stalks in late summer, dry, and store in a jar. When needed, soak the seeds in a small amount of boiling water to form a gel. Apply directly to sore, itchy, or inflamed skin.

❦ For poison ivy, make a tea of decocted sweet fern using the fragrant leaves and flower tops. For a severe case, make a compress and bind it on, changing it as necessary to keep it wet. The tea will stain clothing, so take care.

❦ "Itch: In one pint of gin, steep of black cherry–tree bark, prickly ash, and yellow dock root, each one ounce, adding half a pint of water; and drink two glasses a day." (LIA)

❦ Make a cream or lotion of calendula or chamomile for mild rashes or itching.

❦ For eczema or persistent itching, add about 10 drops each tincture of goldenseal and tincture of dandelion and 5 to 7 drops each tincture of burdock root and tincture of queen's-root to ½ cup water. Make a test on an unaffected patch of skin to be sure these ingredients won't irritate you. If clear, apply to the rash.

❦ For eczema, make a skin cream using true licorice (*Glycyrrhiza uralensis,* from China, or *G. glabra,* from the Mediterranean), which contains glycyrrhizic acid. (**Caution!** Avoid licorice if you have a history of high blood pressure, rapid heart rate, or kidney disease, or if you are pregnant.)

❦ For eczema, massage the area with almond oil, lemon balm oil, or primrose oil. Aloe can alleviate a severely

affected area. A tea made of a decoction of burdock root, red clover, purple coneflower, chamomile, yarrow, or stinging nettles also is helpful.

❦ Native Americans made an ointment of mountain laurel leaves and fat to relieve itching. For spider bites, they used a poultice of mashed balsamroot or tobacco.

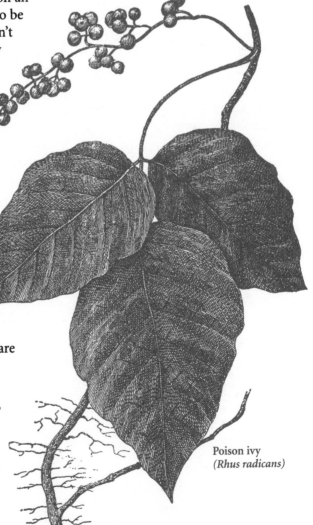

Poison ivy
(*Rhus radicans*)

BURNS & SUNBURNS

Blistered or open burns should never be dressed with any ointment, oil, or salve. Never apply butter or grease to an open burn, for it will expose the wound to contamination and infection. The following remedies are intended for minor burns and sunburns where the skin is red and sore but not blistered or broken. As always, prevention is the best medicine.

❦ "If you get a sunburn, restore your energy with salt tablets or hot tea, which will pep you up and cool you off as well as or better than a cold drink." (OFA, 1945)

❦ "A simple and harmless remedy for a sunburn is to bathe the face in buttermilk." (OFA, 1898)

❦ Wash gently with soap and water and then apply the gel of an older aloe leaf, splitting a leaf open lengthwise for the quantity required.

❦ Apply a mild infusion of purple coneflower to destroy bacteria and soothe the skin.

❦ Grate potatoes and apply to sunburned skin. The starch will cool and soothe the burn.

❦ Apply peppermint oil to sunburned skin, as long as the skin is not broken or blistered. Use a peppermint infusion as a milder wash to help cool a sunburn.

❦ Use apple cider vinegar, plain or diluted, to ease a sunburn.

❦ Make an ointment or salve with the essential oil of Saint Johnswort to promote the healing of burns that have not broken the skin. It is not only anti-inflammatory but also antiviral and antibacterial.

❦ Apply ice or cold water.

Calendula Salve

freshly dried calendula flowers
olive oil

beeswax
benzoin tincture

Chop the dried flowers and cover them with olive oil. Cover and soak for about 2 weeks. Strain through muslin, composting the plant parts, and add up to 4 parts beeswax to every 10 parts calendula oil. A few drops of benzoin tincture will help the salve keep well over time. Store in a covered container. Apply externally to sunburns, minor scrapes and bruises, or chapped lips.

Calendula (*Calendula officinalis*)

❧ Dissolve Epsom salts or baking soda in water, apply to a clean cloth, and drape the cloth over the affected skin.

❧ "For a burn or scald: Immediately plunge the part in cold water: keep it in an hour if not [more]. Perhaps four or five hours. Or, a bruised onion. Or, apply oil and strew on it powdered ginger." (JW)

❧ Take a cool bath, adding lavender or bergamot oil to the bath water.

❧ Mix 1 cup water and 20 to 25 drops lavender oil and use to bathe the sunburned area. Or apply the solution with a spray bottle.

❧ Make an infusion of cooling peppermint or spearmint tea. Drink it and use it to bathe the affected area.

❧ Apply a poultice of dock leaves and water.

❧ Bathe the sunburn with an infusion of stinging nettles, chamomile, or calendula.

❧ Apply aloe or plain yogurt with live cultures.

❧ Native Americans infused ground yarrow in water and used it as a wash.

❧ Wash with an infusion of elder flowers or chickweed.

❧ Apply a compress of decocted witch hazel.

❧ "For a Burn: Take common alum, beat and sift it, and beat it up with whites of eggs to a curd; then with a feather [anoint] the place; it will cure without any other thing." (ES)

TOOTHACHES & CANKER SORES

❧ Chew prickly ash bark.

❧ Apply allspice oil or clove oil to the tooth (but don't swallow it) for pain relief and as an antiseptic. (**Caution!** Clove oil stings.) According to the doctrine of signatures, the shape of the whole clove, resembling a tooth, fitted it for curing toothaches.

❧ Drink chamomile tea.

❧ Use cinnamon toothpaste for its antiseptic qualities, to kill bacteria, fungi, and viruses.

❧ Native Americans applied the mashed green leaves or roots of the willow as a poultice to a toothache.

❧ Press the oil from the thyme plant and apply it to the tooth.

❧ For a toothache, use purple coneflower for its anesthetic properties.

❧ "A Powder for the Teeth: Take half an ounce of cream of tartar, and a quarter of an ounce of powder of myrrh; rub the teeth with it

two or three times a week." (ES)

❦ Make a mouthwash of vinegar and salt to ease toothache pain.

❦ Apply pepper and ginger to a piece of gauze and pack the tooth with it.

❦ Make an infusion of yarrow, hops, peppermint, or dill to ease a toothache.

❦ "Lay bruised or boiled nettles to the cheek. Or, lay a clove of garlic on the tooth. Or, lay a slice of apple lightly boiled between the teeth. Or, keep the feet in warm water, and rub them well with bran just before bed time." (JW)

❦ "To Keep Teeth White: Dip a little piece of white cloth in Vinegar of Quinces, and rub your gums with it, for it is of a gallant binding quality, and not only makes the teeth white, but also strengthens the gums, fastens the teeth, and also causeth a sweet breath." (NC)

❦ "For the Tooth-ache: Take the inner rind of an Elder-tree, and bruise it, and put thereto a little Pepper, and make it into balls, and hold them between the teeth that ache." (NC)

> *Every tooth in a man's head is more valuable than a diamond.*
>
> — MIGUEL DE CERVANTES (1547–1616))

❦ "Make an extract from white poplar bark; mix with it a little rum; put into your tooth, and you will soon find relief." (LIA)

❦ To prevent and treat canker sores, eat plain or vanilla yogurt that contains active cultures. Or, take yogurt tablets, which may be more immediately effective for treating existing sores.

❦ Drink an infusion of lady's-mantle to soothe canker sores.

❦ Avoid orange juice, lemon juice, grapefruit juice, and walnuts if you find yourself prone to canker sores. Drink purple coneflower tea to build up your immunity.

❦ Increase your B complex vitamins to help prevent canker sores.

❦ Apply a pinch of alum directly to the canker sore. It will sting briefly and make you salivate. Try to keep the area relatively dry. Leave on for about a minute, then rinse your mouth with water. This will relieve the pain and make the canker go away faster than it otherwise might. Repeat as necessary once or twice a day.

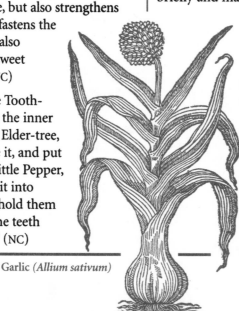

Garlic (*Allium sativum*)

HICCUPS

🐛 Apply ice cubes to either side of the larynx until the hiccups cease.

🐛 Take a spoonful of peanut butter, vinegar, or sugar.

🐛 Suck on ice cubes.

🐛 Eat something very hot and spicy, such as a hot pepper.

🐛 Breathe through a pillow.

🐛 Hold the opening of a paper bag tightly in your fist and cover your mouth, making sure no air can escape. Breathe into it until the hiccups stop.

🐛 "Take three or four preserved damsons in your mouth at a time, and swallow them by degrees." (ES)

🐛 Drink a glass of water from the wrong side of the glass.

🐛 "Swallow a mouthful of water, stopping the mouth and ears. Or, take anything that will make you sneeze. Or, three drops of oil of cinnamon on a lump of sugar." (JW)

🐛 "Take five drops of the oil of amber in mint tea, every ten minutes, until they cease." (LIA)

🐛 Anise seed tea or anise seed eaten dry "helpeth the yeoxing or hicket [hiccups]." (JG)

🐛 Take dill, boil it with wine, then tie it into a rag. Smell it until your yexing [hiccupping] is cured.

WARTS

Warts are contagious. Those occurring on the feet, sometimes called verrucae or plantar warts, are easily picked up if you walk barefoot in public bathrooms, in locker rooms, near swimming pools, or in other public places that remain moist underfoot. Shower sandals and frequent drying of the feet will aid prevention.

🐛 A tea made of purple coneflower, burdock root, or red clover may build up your natural resistance.

🐛 "Rub them daily with a radish. Or, with juice of marigold flowers. It will hardly fail. Or, apply bruised [purslane] as a poultice, changing it twice a day. It cures in seven or eight days." (JW)

🐛 Rub warts with castor oil, lemon juice, macerated dandelion, fresh mashed garlic, celandine juice, or milkweed juice.

🐛 "Warts: Dissolve as much common washing soda as the water will take up, then wash the hands or warts with this for a minute or two, and allow them to dry without being wiped. This repeated for two or three days, will gradually destroy the most irritable wart." (LIA)

Chapter 4

Elixirs, Tonics & Aphrodisiacs

Fill me with sassafras, nurse,
And juniper juice!
Let me see if I'm still any use!
— *DONALD ROBERT PERRY MARQUIS (1878–1937)*

Juniper
(Juniperus communis)

efore we get into elixirs — generally sweetened, medicinal liquids, often containing alcohol — let's talk about water. Long a symbol of fertility, water has been viewed as the substance surrounding the first seeds of life. At baptisms and christenings, water represents new life or rebirth. Some people consider the water bowl or vessel a symbol of womanhood or fertility. Holy wells, magic springs, and water cures have ancient associations with cleansing rituals, healing, longevity, and worship in virtually every culture.

46

In *Primitive Remedies* (1776), John Wesley quotes the "Plain Easy Rules" of his colleague Dr. Cheyne: "Water is the wholesomest of all drinks; it quickens the appetite and strengthens the digestion most." Wesley thought babies should be dipped in cold water every morning until they reached nine months of age to prevent rickets. Furthermore, he prescribed drinking water for "hooping cough," "heartburning," and to prevent kidney stones.

Mrs. Beeton (*Book of Household Management,* 1861) recommended warm water as "preferable to cold water, as a drink, to persons who are subject to dyspeptic [abdominal pains and heartburn] and bilious complaints, and it may be taken more freely than cold water...." In colonial America, "taking the waters" meant either swilling great quantities of mineral spring waters, sold in various forms as patent medicines, or seeking out the spas (alkaline, saline, and sulfur pools, some of them hot), where one could be immersed in the restorative waters reputed to cure nervous, digestive, respiratory, and rheumatic disorders, as well as skin complaints and "general debility."

৵০৻

A voice came o'er the waters far:
"Just drop your bucket where you are."
And then they dipped and drank their fill
Of water fresh from mead and hill.

— SAM WALTER FOSS (1858–1911)

৵০৻

WATER, WATER EVERYWHERE

❦ To aid a reducing diet and/or enhance digestion, drink at least 12 ounces of water with every meal.

❦ To treat brittle nails, drink more water, about six to eight glasses a day, to retain proper moisture levels in the nails and reduce flaking. However, an excess of external water (dishwashing, bathing, wet gardening, and so on) can make brittle nails worse. Wear rubber gloves or coat the nails with petroleum jelly whenever possible.

❦ For urinary tract infections or mild cystitis, increase your water consumption to two to four quarts per day. This is most easily accomplished by drinking a juice glass of water every half hour or so rather than larger amounts less frequently.

❦ To reduce odorous perspiration, drink more water.

❦ According to Dr. N. G. Hunt and his English colleagues (*Lancet,* March 8, 1975), plunging the face in 65° F water often produces a "diving reflex" after 20 to 30 seconds of immersion, in which the heartbeat is dramatically reduced. This diving reflex can be helpful for people who suffer from tachycardia (periodic attacks of rapid heartbeat). (**Caution!** Because there are various types and causes of tachycardia, patients should consult their doctors first.)

❦ To improve your complexion and skin tone and normalize either dry or oily skin, eat well and drink six to eight glasses of water a day.

❦ "The water-cure method of getting rid of coughs and colds is to wrap the body up in a hot, wet sheet, until perspiration is induced, drinking all the time plenty of cold water." (LIA)

❦ "For a cold, drink a pint of cold water lying down in bed." (JW)

❦ "For heartburn, drink a pint of cold water." (JW)

❦ "For a violent case of nosebleed, go into a pond or river." (JW)

❦ "Generally, where cold bathing is necessary to cure any disease, water drinking is so to prevent a relapse." (JW)

❧∽

Here's that which is too weak to be a sinner, —
honest water, which ne'er left man i' the mire.

— WILLIAM SHAKESPEARE (1564–1616)

❧∽

Elixirs

The Compleat Housewife, or Accomplish'd Gentlewoman's Companion (1753) lists various "cordial waters" and their recipes, which brings us to the subject of elixirs. Common ingredients in elixirs, besides alcohols such as brandy, gin, and whiskey, include lemon juice, rhubarb, cream of tartar, Epsom salts, fruit and berry juices, any number of herbs, sweeteners such as molasses and loaf sugar, and various seeds (anise), nuts (walnuts), and roots (horseradish). Less common ingredients are snails, lime, opium, and other medicinals.

To the pharmacist, an elixir is essentially an aromatic, sweetened tincture. That is, the active ingredients of an herb are made soluble with alcohol. That's your tincture. Then scent and sweetener, and perhaps water, are added, and you have an elixir. More than soothing scents, aromatics are antiseptic in nature, contributing more than one might expect to the elixir. *The Ladies Almanac* of 1854 listed a spiced blackberry syrup, used for "summer complaint" (probably a cold and fever), that fits this description. It was made with nutmeg, cloves, and allspice boiled with blackberry juice and sugar. Once it was cool, brandy was added, and the concoction was bottled for future use. It was administered by the teaspoon.

Lemonade, flavored water, switchel or switzel (usually made with ginger and served during haying season), sarsaparilla, Moxie, hot ginger tea, and hot buttered rum all fall under the category of elixirs. Some are meant to be used externally as well as internally. They may be served hot or cold, with or without alcohol, and some rely chiefly on aromatic ingredients inhaled in their steam. Today our healthful elixirs might be the hot toddy for a cough or cold; the early-morning "invigorator" called Bloody Mary, with its tomato juice, celery, and pepper; or the nonalcoholic carrot juice at the gym or fancy bottled water ordered instead of wine.

Blackberry
(*Rubus* spp.)

APPLE CIDER VINEGAR ELIXIRS

Apple cider vinegar may be the number one common denominator among elixir and tonic ingredients. In 1958, practically an entire book was devoted to the benefits of apple cider vinegar as a remedy. Dr. D. C. Jarvis wrote the book, called *Folk Medicine* (Holt, Rinehart and Winston, Inc., 1958), and about half a million copies were sold in the 1960s, as readers sought the "down-to-earth horse sense" of the Vermont doctor, who espoused apple cider vinegar, honey, iodine, kelp, and cod liver oil for most of what ails you. Potassium seems to be the magic component in vinegar. Some people still sip vinegar, in some form, with a meal or just after, for its digestive properties. Applied externally to the skin, it has antiseptic value.

John Parkinson (c. 1640) recommended apple juice and the distilled water of apples for melancholy. Mrs. Beeton identified wine vinegar as a Roman cure, considered to be "digestive, antibilious, and antiscorbutic [preventing scurvy], as well as refreshing."

❦ "Wash the temples, nose, and neck with vinegar to stop a nosebleed. Or, snuff vinegar up the nose. Or, burn a vinegar-soaked rag and sniff the smoke (also good for lethargy)." (JW)

❦ "Make a compress of a pint of vinegar and an ounce of alum and apply to the temples to ease a nosebleed. Steep the feet in warm water." (JW)

❦ Apply a compress of vinegar and water to the temples to ease a violent headache.

❦ Make a poultice of white wine, vinegar, and bran and apply to a sprain.

❦ "Take a glass of vinegar for a fit of indigestion." (JW)

❦ Pour ¼ cup apple cider vinegar into a mug, add 1 tablespoon honey, and fill with boiling water. Drink at mealtimes to aid digestion or before bed to ease insomnia. This is a good, all-purpose tonic for stomach ills, for skin problems, and to maintain proper weight.

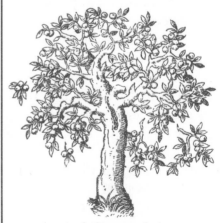

Apple (*Pyrus malus*)

LEMON ELIXIRS

"The lemon," says Mrs. Beeton, "makes one of our most popular and refreshing beverages — lemonade, which is gently stimulating and cooling, and soon quenches the thirst. But, persons with irritable stomachs should avoid it, on account of its acid qualities."

❦ For a cough, "make a hole through a lemon and fill it with honey. Roast it and catch the juice. Take a teaspoon of this frequently." (JW)

❦ For an intermittent fever, "drink warm lemonade in the beginning of every fit; it cures in a few days." (JW)

❦ For a headache, "apply to each temple the thin yellow rind of a lemon newly pared off. Or, pour upon the palm of the hand a little brandy and some zest of lemon, and hold it to the forehead."(JW)

❦ For digestion, "drink the juice of half a large lemon, or sweet orange, immediately after dinner every day." (JW)

❦ "For a refreshing summer drink, take 2 pounds loaf sugar, 2 pints water, 1 ounce citric acid, and ½ drachm essence of lemon. Boil the sugar and water together for ¼ hour, put it in a basin, and let it remain there till cold. Beat the citric acid to a powder, mix the essence of lemon with it, and add these two ingredients to the syrup; mix well and bottle for use. Two tablespoons of the syrup are sufficient for a tumbler of water." (MB)

❦ Make a syrup of lemon rind to reduce a fever or for use as a gargle or sore throat. Mixed with cinnamon, it reduces the likelihood of vomiting caused by fever.

Nourishing Lemonade

rind of 2 lemons
6 ounces loaf sugar
1½ pints boiling water

½ pint sherry
juice of 4 lemons
4 eggs, well beaten and strained

"Pare off the lemon rind thinly, put it in a jug with the sugar, and pour over the boiling water. Let it cool, then strain it; add the sherry, lemon juice, and eggs, and the beverage will be ready for use. If thought desirable, the quantity of sherry and water could be lessened, and milk substituted for them. To obtain the flavour of the lemon-rind properly, a few lumps of sugar should be rubbed over it, until some of the yellow is absorbed."   From Mrs. Beeton's *Book of Household Management*, 1861.

GINGER & OTHER ELIXIRS

❦ Ginger Tea: For feverish colds, discomfort with the menses, or diarrhea, make an infusion of 1 teaspoon ground ginger in 1 pint boiling water. Strain. Add lemon and brown sugar or honey.

❦ Switchel, or switzel: 4 cups sugar (or other sweetener such as molasses, brown sugar, maple syrup, or honey), 1 cup vinegar, 2 tablespoons ground ginger, 2 gallons water. Mix together the first 3 ingredients, then add the water and refrigerate until very cold. Serve at haying time or during any hot work under the sun.

❦ Quick Ginger Beer: Dissolve 4 ounces candied ginger in 2 gallons boiling water. Add 2 pounds sugar, ¼ ounce citric acid, and 2 tablespoons yeast. Let stand for at least 24 hours, strain, and bottle. Let age for at least 1 week, longer if possible.

❦ Haying Cooler: Take a gallon of water and add enough cream of tartar to make it look cloudy. Sweeten as you like and drink cold.

❦ Mint Refresher: Boil together 1 pound sugar and 1 quart water. Meanwhile, chop 1 to 2 cups mint leaves very fine, then grind with a mortar and pestle, adding about ¼ cup sugar to the grinding process. Once the boiled sugar water has cooled slightly, add the mint mixture and the juice of 3 to 5 lemons. Refrigerate until ice-cold and serve on a hot day. For a cold or cough, heat and serve with bourbon or other alcohol of your choice.

❦ Pepper Tea: Put 1 teaspoon black pepper and 1 teaspoon sugar in a mug. Pour in boiling water and let steep. The pepper will settle to the bottom. Sip to suppress a night cough.

❦ Honey and Sherry: Heat ¼ cup good sherry. Put 1 teaspoon honey in a mug, add the sherry, and fill with boiling water. Sprinkle nutmeg over the top. This is a good winter warm-up and promotes relaxation and sleep.

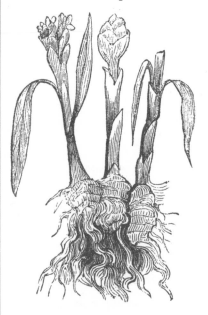

Ginger (*Zingiber officinalis*)

❦ Summer Complaint Cordial: Steep ½ ounce pulverized rhubarb and ½ ounce baking soda in ½ pint water for 30 minutes. Add ½ pound sugar and simmer until dissolved. Strain and add ½ ounce chopped peppermint leaves and 4 ounces brandy. Bottle. Take by the teaspoonful every 2 to 3 hours until the fever is gone.

❦ Balsamum Vitae, or "Balsam of Life" (a restorative in vogue in the early 1800s and prescribed in various recipes): Combine ¼ ounce each oil of lavender, oil of cloves, oil of lemon, and oil of cinnamon; 6 drops rose water; and 1 pint alcohol such as vodka or gin. The dose is 1 teaspoon, taken on a lump of sugar, sometimes dropped into a glass of sherry or Madeira, and occasionally beaten with an egg yolk.

❦ Cinnamon Cordial: Pour a bottle of good Cognac on 3 ounces bruised (ground) cinnamon. Take by the spoonful. Especially helpful for students and to increase memory.

Steaming Bishop

1 navel orange
whole cloves

¼ cup maple syrup
1 bottle good red Burgundy

Stud the orange with the cloves and roast at 350° F for 30 minutes. Cut into quarters, put in a saucepan, and add the maple syrup and Burgundy. Heat on low just until the wine begins to steam. Serve in mugs. For a more warming drink, add ½ cup brandy just before serving. Good for colds and flu.

Orange (*Citrus sinensis*)

Spring Tonics

If you think back to what was on the menu during the long, cold, dark winters of colonial America, you quickly get a picture of why spring tonics were important. After all those potatoes, cabbages, winter squashes, and various root vegetables that sustained the early settlers, something a little green, a bit purging, and altogether different was definitely in order by early spring. Dandelion greens, asparagus, early cresses, thistles, burdock (root and/or aerial parts), stinging nettles, purslane, lamb's quarters, parsley, violet leaves, curly dock (yellow dock), sheep sorrel, spinach, and plantain were among the early risers of spring, bringing their longed-for greenery and treasure-trove of vitamins and minerals back to the dinner table. As potherbs, they were boiled or steamed; buttered; sprinkled with bacon bits, vinegar, or lemon juice; or otherwise dressed up. Just plain, they made salads where there had been none before.

As kitchen medicines, these spring tonic ingredients are largely diuretic. Just as the colonial housewife prepared for the great spring cleaning of the household, so too did she commence to purge the family's winter-dulled digestive systems. Good riddance to scurvy! The spring tonic herbs brought new sources of vitamin A and carotene, vitamin C and antioxidants, calcium, iron, and fiber. A splash of vinegar added a little extra potassium.

Other spring tonics took the form of the sulfur and molasses, or blackstrap molasses, concoctions, which, quite literally, had the physical effect of a spring cleaning. Highly laxative and often causing malodorous gas attacks, a sulfur and molasses remedy was probably the spring tonic version of winter's cod liver oil.

Burdock (*Arctium* spp.)

DANDELIONS

Once prized as a diuretic, tonic, and aperient, for "derangement of digestive organs" and dropsical afflictions, the common dandelion was the spring tonic ingredient of choice. It contains vitamins A, B, C, and D, as well as iron and potassium, and is certainly a welcome early-spring green.

John Gerard's *Herball* (1597) recommends the dandelion to cure incontinence and to open and cleanse the system. Eaten raw, Gerard said, it "stops the bellie and helps the Dysentery." Dandelion juice, boiled with vinegar, was a bladder remedy. Nicholas Culpeper (1652) said it would remedy ague fits.

As children, we learned to suck the milky juice from dandelion stems, and we considered it a "survival secret" in case we were in need of fluids. In fact, too much of this juice can make a child sick with vomiting or diarrhea and should be especially discouraged where lawns are treated with chemicals. Let the kids use the milky juices to get rid of warts instead.

❦ For a cleansing spring tonic, eat young dandelion greens raw or cooked like beet greens or spinach.

❦ Spring Tonic: Take up the roots, clean them, bruise in a mortar, and press out the juice. Strain the juice and put on a plate in a warm room to render it thick and solid. Dose: a scruple to a drachm three times a day.

❦ Eat dandelion greens as a detoxifier of the liver, kidneys, blood, and tissues after a long winter of heavy, fatty foods; after cancer treatments or other extreme drug therapies; after an overindulgence in alcohol, sweets, or fats; or after jaundice, hepatitis, or gallbladder infections.

❦ Use a tincture or decoction of dandelion roots (best harvested in the fall) for gout, eczema, and acne.

❦ Eat dandelion greens to help prevent urinary tract infections.

❦ Take decocted dandelion roots as a gentle laxative.

❦ Drink an infusion of dandelion greens and flowers as a calming tea.

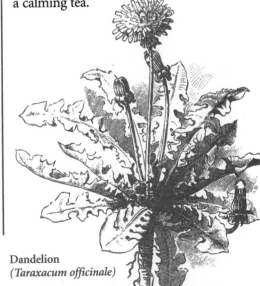

Dandelion
(*Taraxacum officinale*)

❦ Native Americans chewed dandelion stems like gum, to moisten the mouth in dusty conditions.

❦ Colonial settlers made a "poke salad" of dandelions, cowslips, cresses, and pigweed for a spring pick-me-up.

❦ For yellow jaundice, Native Americans used dandelion bitters (from the root).

❦ For heart trouble, some Native American tribes boiled new dandelion flowers in water until the water turned yellow, then cooled it overnight and drank it every morning for a month.

❦ Native Americans also decocted dandelions to use in treating hypochondria.

❦ For a relaxing body rub, soak equal parts finely chopped dandelions, burdock (root and/or aerial parts), yellow dock, and lobelia in 1 quart rubbing alcohol for at least 2 weeks.

❦ For swelling and sores, make a poultice of dandelions.

❦ To remove warts, pick dandelions two or three times a day and rub the milky juice from the stems on the warts.

The Wonderful Weed

Young Leaves (gathered before the plant blooms): Use in tossed and wilted salads, either alone or in combination with other wild greens or garden vegetables. Young dandelion leaves are tangy and very nutritious. They make a tasty potherb when cooked like spinach, or they may be added to a pot of mixed greens.

Roots: When digging dandelions for greens, save the roots to roast and grind for a coffeelike beverage or to add to ground coffee in the way that chicory is used. Scrub the dandelion roots, drain, and place on a baking sheet. Roast at 150° F for about four hours, or until the roots are dark and dry. Cool and then grind the roots in a food grinder or blender. Store in a covered jar.

Dried Leaves: Use for tea.

Flowers: Use for making wine, edible garnishes, and jelly. Deep-fry the flowers to make a delicious snack or hors d'oeuvre that tastes a little like a morel prepared the same way.

From "The Dandelion — A Wonderful Weed with Dozens of Uses" by Marilyn Kluger, *The Old Farmer's Almanac*, 1977.

"Dent-de-Lioun" Wine

The Middle English name dent-de-lioun *comes from the Medieval Latin* dens leonis, *which means "lion's tooth" and may allude to the sharply indented toothlike leaves of the plant.*

2 quarts dandelion petals
4 quarts water
2 oranges, cut into small pieces
2 lemons, cut into small pieces
1 cake yeast
3½ pounds sugar

Pick the dandelions early in the morning, gathering enough flower heads to make 2 quarts of petals after the stem and green collar at the end of each flower have been snipped off. Rinse the dandelions in cool water before preparing the petals.

Place the dandelion petals in a large nonreactive pan and cover with the water. Boil for 20 minutes. Pour the hot liquid and petals over the orange and lemon pieces. Allow the mixture to cool to lukewarm. Add the yeast and let stand for 48 hours. Strain the mixture through cheesecloth, squeezing to remove all the juice. Add the sugar to the juice and stir well to dissolve.

Pour the liquid into a jug, such as a glass cider jug. Cover with a lid but do *not* screw the cap down tightly. Or close with a water seal: use a cork with a tube inserted through it for the stopper and put the other end of the tube into a glass of water. Let the wine stand for about 6 weeks, or until still. Strain and bottle. Keep for at least 6 months before drinking, as this wine improves with age. Makes about 5 four-fifths wine bottles.

From "The Dandelion — A Wonderful Weed with Dozens of Uses" by Marilyn Kluger, *The Old Farmer's Almanac*, 1977.

Other Tonics

The Civil War tonic was used to restore the spirits, cure coughs, and increase morale — whether Union or Confederate! The ingredients were ground ginger, sugar, red currants, lemon juice, and good whiskey. The dosage was unspecified, but we suspect that this tonic was carefully rationed according to the supply.

Shipboard rum rations, vinegar and water for the Roman army, and wine vinegar with salt in water for the Spanish peasantry all share a common bond with this Civil War tonic. Whether restorative to morale, used as a physic, or helping to reduce contagious diseases, all were tonic remedies. Similarly, Coca-Cola was originally a medicinal tonic containing cocaine. It was advertised as a brain tonic and to ease the menses. Sarsaparilla, commonly sipped as a soda pop until recently, was first a decoction of the roots of the sarsaparilla plant that was made into various tonics reputed to be medicinal. John Gerard recommended sarsaparilla for rheumatism and colds.

Sarsaparilla (*Smilax aspera*)

CIDER

Cider, which used to mean the hard, alcoholic version from fermented apple juice, was another digestive aid, used primarily in the autumn and winter months and sometimes mixed with rum and spices or raisins as mulled or spiced cider. "Stone wall" was the name of one such rum and cider tonic, which was sometimes sweetened with brown sugar. It was a reputed remedy for chills.

Apple brandy and applejack are other versions of cider with an even higher alcohol content. These were sometimes added to cough remedies.

Sweet cider (unfermented) was available only during the apple harvest. It was served hot and spiced to ward off colds and flu.

❦ Apple syrup "is a good cordial in faintings, palpitations, and melancholy." (NC)

❦ Eat fresh apples or drink apple juice or cider for constipation.

❦ Make a poultice of stewed, whole apples for skin afflictions and rheumatism.

❦ Use cider and apple juice as natural antiseptics.

❦ Eat stewed apples to cure diarrhea.

❦ Take unsweetened apple juice, cider, or raw apples for urinary tract infections and cystitis. Taken warm, they can ease stomach colic and feverish colds.

Mulled Cider

4 cups sweet cider
½ teaspoon ground cinnamon
¼ teaspoon ground nutmeg
pinch of ground cloves
brown sugar (optional)
dark rum (optional)

Combine the cider with the cinnamon, nutmeg, and cloves. Sweeten with the brown sugar if desired. Heat to steaming (don't boil). Serve as is or add dark rum to ward off winter chills and colds.

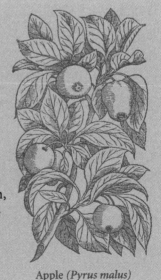

Apple *(Pyrus malus)*

Aphrodisiacs

Dr. Cheyne, quoted by John Wesley in his 18th-century book, listed as the second of his "Plain Easy Rules" (after breathing good air) that "tender people should have those who lie with them, or are much about them, sound, sweet, and healthy." Once you have that problem solved, you can proceed to what is often described in the remedy books as a matter of "vigor."

For starters, Perdita, in William Shakespeare's *The Winter's Tale,* suggests "hot lavender, mints, savory, marjoram…given to men of middle age." Rosemary and thyme have been combined, at least in myth, to effect a seduction, and lavender strewn among the linens is surely much more than a mere moth repellent. Garlic, which, in the language and sentiment of flowers, says "I can't stand you," seems to be a two-faced herb, as the Greeks considered it among their aphrodisiacs, probably for its reputation for increasing a man's strength and endurance. We presume that Aphrodite intended both partners to consume it, perhaps followed by parsley, also a Greek herb of love and known to sweeten the breath.

PASSION BOOSTERS

❦ "Artichokes open obstructions, provoke urination, produce wind, warm the viscera, increase coitus and make the member stiff." (ITALIAN FOLKLORE, C. 1500)

❦ Orchids take their name from the genus *Orchis,* which comes from the Greek word for testicle, because of the resemblance of the plant's fleshy roots to that male part. Remedies have included eating the flower to aid fertility.

❦ The tomato, once considered poisonous to eat, also was reputed to stir lust if consumed in small doses.

❦ Anise seed "allayeth gripings of the belly, provoketh urine gently, maketh aboundance of milke, and stirreth up bodily lust." (JG)

❦ Burdock root, eaten raw, was supposed to "increaseth seed and stirreth up lust." (JG)

❦ Myrtle leaves "eaten by man and wife together causeth love between them." (NC)

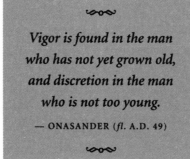

Vigor is found in the man who has not yet grown old, and discretion in the man who is not too young.

— ONASANDER (*fl.* A.D. 49)

❦ "In all cases, avoid constipation, the hand maiden of impotence and derangement." (Dr. Frederick Hollick, c. 1840) Eat prunes or drink prune juice to avoid constipation.

❦ For a high sperm count, keep your zinc levels high. Foods high in zinc include oysters, lean beef, crabmeat, cowpeas, lentils, clams, lobster, lima beans, and dark turkey meat.

❦ Enjoy seafood such as oysters, lobster, mussels, clams, caviar, and herring.

❦ Heed the doctrine of signatures and choose foods resembling the sex organs, such as carrots, asparagus, cucumbers, bananas, mandrake root, wild yam root, ginseng, gingerroot, garlic, and figs.

❦ Drink dandelion juice to prevent "the involuntary effusion of seed." (JG)

❦ Make an herb oil or salve of ginger and use it to massage the lower back to bring heat to that area and increase the circulation.

❦ Before nuptials, drink an infusion of celery. Or, mix a pulverized head of celery with a good French white wine, let sit for 2 days, strain, and drink a glass a day for a week.

❦ Use rose water, rose bath oil, or rose massage oil as a stimulant for women.

❦ Mix basil or savory with wine (an ounce of dried herbs to a bottle of good wine, port, or Madeira) and drink a glassful before a romantic evening.

❦ Eat or drink chocolate in moderation. The Aztec emperor Montezuma swore by it as a virility booster.

❦ Drink ginseng tea at bedtime for vigor.

Endurance-Maker Lemon Cocktail

juice of 1 lemon
2 tablespoons water
3 tablespoons powdered milk
1 tablespoon honey, or more to taste

Combine all the ingredients, stir vigorously, and consume. Two of these cocktails a day, as a regular habit, is the recommended dose.

Chapter 5

Food for Health & Well-Being

Dyspepsy is the ruin of most things:
empires, expeditions, and
everything else.

— *THOMAS DE QUINCY (1785–1862)*

The remarkable thing about most early "receipt" books (cookbooks) is that they were an informal compendium of food recipes — such as family wedding cakes, meat pies, and jellies — and formulas for natural remedies made from various foods and herbs, including cough drops, spring tonics, chest plasters, and other cures. The books might have been used as diaries and account books as well, the front pages for one purpose, the back for another. Sometimes even-numbered pages contained recipes, then

Peppermint
(Mentha × piperita)

the book was turned upside down, and ongoing financial accounts were recorded on odd-numbered pages.

Generally, sources of recipes were credited, whether family member, neighbor, or friend. A new pastor might pass on remedies from his former parish or from working closely with a certain doctor. Indian cures were not unusual, gleaned by way of trading posts or even from former captives who had returned to their villages. Newspapers and church newsletters were other sources of recipes and remedies.

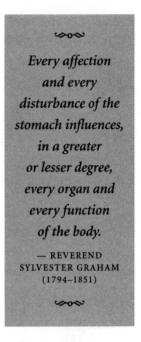

Every affection and every disturbance of the stomach influences, in a greater or lesser degree, every organ and every function of the body.

— REVEREND SYLVESTER GRAHAM (1794–1851)

Remedies for Digestive Troubles

Many of the recipes collected in early cookbooks were both food and medicine. These might be preventive in nature, curative, or both.

A balanced diet is key to proper digestion. Eating a variety of foods, including plenty of vegetables, fruits, and whole-grain products, will help you achieve a healthy balance. An upset of that balance can lead to dyspepsia, heartburn, indigestion, diarrhea, or constipation.

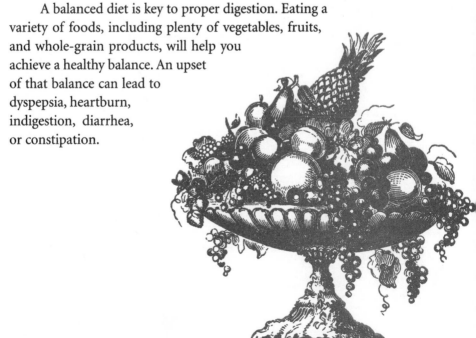

DYSPEPSIA & HEARTBURN

Old recipe books often speak of dyspepsia, offering, for example, a recipe for dyspepsia bread. Dyspepsia covers a multitude of symptoms that may include heartburn, belching, a bloated or gassy feeling in the stomach, indigestion, and abdominal pain. Stress and diet can affect it.

❦ "Drink a pint of cold water. Or, drink slowly a decoction of camomile flowers. Or, eat four or five oysters. Or, chew five or six pepper corns a little, then swallow them. Or, chew fennel or parsley, and swallow your spittle." (JW)

❦ For heartburn, drink a glass of water with a teaspoon of baking soda dissolved in it.

❦ For preventing heartburn, cook with herbs such as basil, bay leaves, caraway, ginger, marjoram, mint, oregano, pepper, savory, and thyme. Eat slowly and at least three hours before bedtime.

❦ To reduce heartburn, avoid cooking in copper or aluminum.

❦ To ease heartburn, drink milk.

❦ To prevent heartburn, drink a glass of water, with a squeeze of lemon juice added, with your meal.

❦ Powdered slippery elm bark in capsule form or mixed with water has been used to treat heartburn. It can be combined with marshmallow root.

Dyspepsia Bread

"Dyspepsia bread" and "Graham bread," named for Reverend Sylvester Graham, were used interchangeably for bread made with whole bran, which was supposed to cure indigestion.

3 quarts unbolted wheat meal [bran]
1 quart soft water, warm but not hot
1 gill [¼ cup] molasses (optional)
1 teaspoon saleratus [baking soda]

Combine the ingredients and form into two loaves. Bake at 400° F for 1 hour.

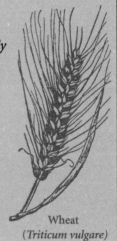

Wheat
(*Triticum vulgare*)

STOMACHACHES

Ginger is probably the number one herb used to prevent indigestion, prevent or cure motion sickness, ward off ulcers, and protect against intestinal parasites. Old advice about ulcers tends to be outdated. For example, doctors no longer recommend drinking milk, which may actually aggravate an ulcer. Additionally, it's unlikely that caffeine or spicy foods cause ulcers, although once you have an ulcer, you may want to avoid them if they irritate your stomach. Salt is still considered a contributing factor, so it's a good idea to cut down on your salt intake. Experiment with foods in your regular diet to find out which ones cause distress. Use polyunsaturated vegetable oil in lieu of other cooking oils as much as possible, as it seems to have a protective effect.

❦ Start to address stomach problems by eliminating alcohol, caffeine, and tobacco.

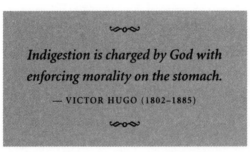

Indigestion is charged by God with enforcing morality on the stomach.

— VICTOR HUGO (1802–1885)

❦ Chamomile, ginger, and peppermint teas are the most widely used herbal infusions for stomach distress. Chamomile flowers are particularly useful and well suited for children's stomach complaints. The more bitter the infusion (flowers left to steep 20 minutes or longer), the more effective it is for indigestion.

❦ Eat yogurt with live cultures to help restore balance to the stomach. Choose unsweetened or vanilla-flavored varieties.

❦ If you experience difficulty with gas or bloating, try adding peppermint, in various forms, to your daily diet. Some studies suggest that peppermint oil is more effective than teas or lozenges.

❦ Anyone traveling to unfamiliar regions and partaking of unusual foods would do well to add ginger to his or her daily diet. Some travelers carry ginger syrup with them, which can be added to hot or cold beverages. (See the section on ginger elixirs in Chapter 4.)

❦ Powdered carob, mixed with yogurt or applesauce, can bring relief from indigestion.

❦ Drink ginger tea, consume it in capsule form, add ground ginger to foods, or indulge in ginger cookies or crystallized ginger candy.

❦ For breast-fed babies with colic, consider whether foods in the mother's diet may be leading to digestive troubles for the infant. The brassicas (cauliflower, cabbage, and Brussels sprouts, for example) are often culprits. Also watch out for alcohol, too much sugar, and caffeine in coffee, soda, tea, and chocolate. Onions, leeks, garlic, peppers, cucumbers, beans, lentils, tomatoes, eggplant, and even eggs can cause upsets. Fruit is generally OK, but eat it in moderation. (See the section on aromatic baths in Chapter 7 for other possible cures for colic.)

Ginger Trio Cookies

These cookies are good to bring on board a ship, for children with a stomachache, or for any other case of an upset stomach.

¾ cup (1½ sticks) butter, softened
1 cup brown sugar
¼ cup molasses
1 egg
2 generous cups flour
2 teaspoons baking soda
1 tablespoon ground ginger

½ teaspoon salt
2 tablespoons finely chopped gingerroot
½ cup finely chopped crystallized ginger

Cream together the butter and sugar. Beat in the molasses and egg. Sift together the flour, baking soda, ground ginger, and salt and add to the butter mixture. Add the gingerroot and crystallized ginger, stirring well. Refrigerate, covered, for at least 2 hours or overnight.

Preheat the oven to 350° F. Drop 1-inch balls of dough onto greased cookie sheets and bake for about 10 minutes. Makes 3 to 4 dozen, depending on size.

DIARRHEA, OR FLUX

We list these remedies as potentially useful for mild stomach and intestinal upsets or to supplement other treatments. Some of the herbs are recommended for both diarrhea and constipation, which may seem contradictory. It is not, however, as some herbs work to restore the balance of the bowels, bringing either extreme back to the norm. (See the section on spring tonics in Chapter 4, which also addresses the subject of balancing the bowels.)

A medical expert should be consulted in any case of continued constipation or diarrhea, especially when blood is present. Infants and young children particularly should get immediate medical attention in such cases.

❦ Foods to prevent or treat diarrhea include bananas, blackberries, milk, raspberries, rhubarb (use in moderation), and tomatoes. Teas made with chamomile, blackberry root bark, marshmallow root, cinnamon bark, lady'smantle, yarrow, agrimony, or raspberry leaves also are helpful.

❦ Herbs for diarrhea include goldenseal, poplar bark, skullcap, cinnamon, ginger, nutmeg, chamomile, and bayberry. Add them to foods or use in teas.

❦ For children with diarrhea, make sure fluid intake is adequate to prevent dehydration. Give the child water or herbal teas (chamomile, ginger, raspberry, or lemon balm) rather than fruit juices. Excessive fruit or fruit juice consumption can be problematic, especially citrus fruits, apples, plums, and strawberries. Feed the child white or brown rice, bananas, rice pudding with cinnamon, or yogurt with cinnamon or honey.

❦ Add a tablespoon of powdered carob to yogurt with active cultures or applesauce to bring relief.

❦ "Drink cold water as largely as possible, taking nothing else till the flux stops. Or, grated rhubarb, as much as lies on a shilling, with half as much grated nutmeg, in a glass of white wine, at lying down every other night. Or, feed on rice, saloup [saloop], sago, and sometimes on beef tea; but no flesh.... A person was cured in one day by feeding on rice milk, and sitting a quarter of an hour in a shallow tub, having in it warm water, three inches deep." (JW)

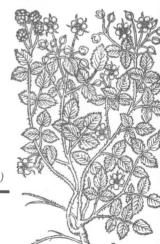

Raspberry
(*Rubus idaeus*)

Rice Pudding

Various recipes for rice pudding are listed in old recipe books, and most are noted for their use in the nursery or for convalescents. As common fare or for bowel regulation, they may include fresh or dried fruits such as currants, raisins, or apples. Rice pudding was probably the most common remedy for children with diarrhea, used so often that many youngsters came to hate it.

1⅓ cups milk
⅛ teaspoon salt
4 to 6 tablespoons granulated sugar or ½ cup brown sugar
1 tablespoon butter, softened
1 teaspoon vanilla or almond extract
2 to 4 eggs
½ teaspoon grated lemon rind
1 teaspoon lemon juice
⅓ cup raisins or other dried fruit
2 cups cooked white rice
cinnamon sugar

Combine the milk, salt, sugar, butter, vanilla or almond extract, and eggs. Beat well. Add the lemon rind, lemon juice, and raisins or other fruit. Stir in the rice. Spread the mixture in a buttered baking dish and bake at 325° F for 50 minutes, or until set. Sprinkle with cinnamon sugar.

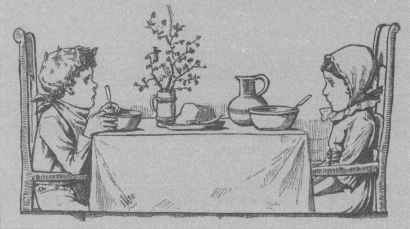

CONSTIPATION, OR COSTIVENESS

Many of the elixirs and spring tonics in Chapter 4 also are useful in helping to balance the bowels and increase natural sources of iron without the complication of constipation.

❦ "Rise early every morning. Or, boil in a pint and a half of broth, half a handful of mallow leaves chopped, strain this and drink it before you eat anything else. Do this frequently, if needful. Or, breakfast twice a week or oftener, on water gruel with currants. Or, take daily, two hours before dinner a small tea cupful of stewed prunes.… Or, live upon bread made of wheat flour with all the bran in it." (JW)

❦ A classic old remedy for constipation is to drink a glass of lemon juice and water first thing in the morning. (**Caution!** This can be hard on teeth enamel, in which case try a teaspoon of honey in hot water every morning.)

❦ Eat a daily serving of yogurt with live cultures to help the balance of good bacteria in the bowels.

❦ Make sure that your daily diet includes garlic, onions, or leeks to encourage a balance of good bacteria.

❦ Herbs to ease constipation include peppermint, goldenseal, and butternut bark.

❦ Sufficient exercise and fluids are key in treating constipation. Exercise speeds the progress of foods through your system, so a simple walk can be helpful. For best results, take a walk at the first signs of difficulty.

❦ Increasing your daily consumption of fiber or bran by just a little may be all the treatment you need. Always increase your water intake with any increase in fiber; otherwise, you run the risk of clogging up your system with all that roughage. Two bran biscuits and

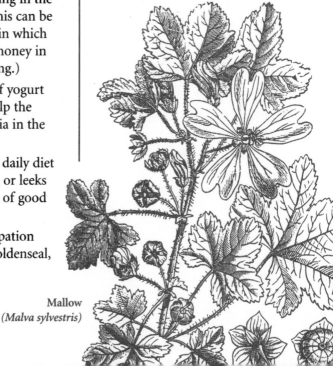

Mallow
(*Malva sylvestris*)

a glass of water, two tablespoons of wheat bran on a cup of yogurt or applesauce, or a bowl of bran cereal with milk may be sufficient.

❧ Rhubarb root, a potent herb, can be used for constipation. (**Caution!** Do not use if pregnant.)

❧ Caffeinated teas and coffees can aggravate a tendency toward constipation, especially during pregnancy. Iron tablets and prenatal vitamins also can promote constipation. Look for natural sources of iron (organic meats, parsley, molasses, or egg yolks, for example). Many of the herbs that are used to treat constipation also contain iron, such as dandelion leaves, burdock root, yellow dock root, and raspberry leaves. Sip a little watered-down apple cider vinegar half an hour before meals to increase your ability to absorb natural iron.

❧ Young children, especially bottle-fed infants, who experience constipation may be showing food intolerances. Try eliminating wheat, cow's milk, refined foods, and sugar. Increase vitamin C and magnesium for older children.

❧ "For Costiveness: Take virgin-honey a quarter of a pound, and mix it with as much cream of tartar as will bring it to a thick electuary, of which take the bigness of a walnut when you please; and for your breakfast eat water-gruel with common mallows boiled in it, and a good piece of butter; the mallows must be chopped small, and eaten with the gruel." (ES)

❧ Foods to prevent and ease constipation include figs (or syrup of figs), prunes, and apricots. Teas also may help, especially the decocted roots of dandelion, yellow dock, angelica, burdock, ginger, and licorice or infusions of fennel, peppermint, chamomile, or raspberry leaves.

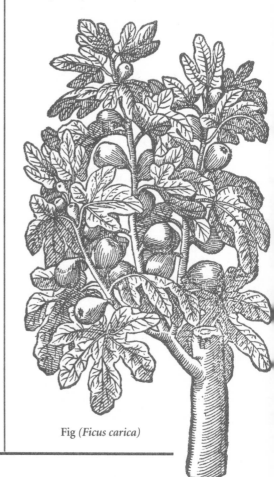

Fig (*Ficus carica*)

Remedies for Urinary Ailments

Did you know that your kidneys filter about 1,000 gallons of fluid a day? Is it any wonder that as we age, our kidneys show signs of distress? Tobacco, alcohol, caffeine (and other stimulants), high blood pressure, diabetes, frequent urinary tract infections, and even strep throat can put our kidneys at greater risk. Pesticides, food additives and preservatives, and other toxins in our food and environment also increase the burden on our kidneys. When it comes to better kidney health, prevention and good diet are key. Flushing the system with sufficient water and other diuretics (substances that act on the kidneys to increase the production of urine) also is helpful.

KIDNEY COMPLAINTS

❦ Never allow yourself to become dehydrated. Drink all the water you can to help flush your system.

❦ Avoid urinary tract infections. Drink cranberry juice (seek organic sources, free of pesticides) and avoid stimulants.

❦ Stay "low on the food chain." Reduce protein consumption dramatically, eating a maximum of two to four ounces of meat a day. Because protein sources are high on the food chain, they're more apt to be contaminated with toxins, and they often contain toxic residues and additives. Thus, digestion of proteins puts unnecessary stress on the liver and kidneys.

❦ Chinese medicine advises increasing the use of salty herbs for kidney and bladder difficulties. Seaweed, dulse, fenugreek, and saw palmetto are some examples.

❦ Add horseradish to your diet to stimulate digestion and enhance the passage of urine. It's one of the more powerful herbal diuretics and can be grated into foods, made into a syrup, or decocted with mustard seed and boiling water for good results.

❦ According to the doctrine of signatures, decocted kidney bean pods are helpful for kidney troubles, including urinary retention and urinary tract infections. The pods must be fresh, however.

❦ Other kidney-enhancing beans include black soybeans and black beans. Cook them with garlic and use them to replace meat proteins. Incidentally, kidney beans are among the best sources of vitamin B_6.

❦ It has been suggested that adequate amounts of magnesium

oxide and vitamin B$_6$ in the diet help prevent kidney troubles. Foods often recommended to enhance normal kidney function include asparagus, artichokes, parsley, parsnips, strawberries, watercress, and watermelon, most of which contain both substances in good amounts.

❦ Medicinal Uses of Asparagus: "This plant not only acts as a wholesome and nutritious vegetable, but also as a diuretic, aperient, and deobstruent." (MB)

❦ The decocted root of the second-year parsley plant has been recommended for dispelling gravel or small stones. The leaves can be infused (not boiled) for similar results. Infuse 1 teaspoon

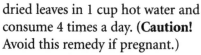

Gravelroot (*Eupatorium purpureum*)

dried leaves in 1 cup hot water and consume 4 times a day. (**Caution!** Avoid this remedy if pregnant.)

❦ Decocted milk thistle seeds and decocted dandelion roots enhance liver function and can help fight hepatitis. They can be taken with Siberian ginseng or angelica.

❦ Chickweed in salads or as an infused tea, burdock root in soups or decocted as a tea, stinging nettle leaves, decocted dandelion roots, and dandelion greens in salads all benefit the kidneys.

❦ Avoid air-conditioned rooms and airplanes, which put added stress on the kidneys.

❦ Gravelroot is a diuretic herb that can be decocted to prevent gravel in the urine.

❦ For kidney stones, eat baked or steamed parsnips every day for a week.

❦ For Stones in the Kidneys: "Use the cold bath. Or, drink half a pint of water every morning. Or, boil an ounce of common thistle-root, and four drachms of liquorice, in a pint of water. Drink of it every morning." (JW)

❦ For Gravel: "Eat largely of spinach. Or, drink largely of warm water sweetened with honey." (JW)

❦ For Sharp Urine: "Take two spoonsful of fresh juice of ground-ivy." (JW)

BED-WETTING & INCONTINENCE

For bed-wetting in children, consider whether anxiety is an issue and what you might do to relieve it. For example, if the child has just changed schools or moved, bed-wetting might commence. Also consider whether the child might have a bladder infection. Never shame a child for bed-wetting; it only makes matters worse.

❦ Administer a teaspoonful of pure honey before bedtime, withholding all liquids after supper.

A human being: an ingenious assembly of portable plumbing.

— CHRISTOPHER MORLEY (1890–1957)

❦ Some children, especially boys between the ages of three and six, may need to be awakened once in the night and brought to the toilet until their bladders are more developed.

❦ Sweet sumac or Saint Johnswort might help. Give it in tincture form with a small amount of water or fruit juice or mixed with honey.

❦ Agrimony, corn silk, shepherd's purse, and mullein have all been recommended for enuresis or bed-wetting.

❦ "For Urine by Drops, with Heat and Pain: Drink nothing but lemonade. Or, beat up the pulp of five or six roasted apples with a quart of water. Use it at lying down. It commonly cures before morning." (JW) (**Caution!** See your doctor.)

❦ "Involuntary Urine: Use the cold bath. Or, take a teaspoonful of powdered agrimony in a little water morning and evening." (JW)

❦ For Suppression of Urine: "Drink largely of warm lemonade." (JW)

❦ Before sleeping, massage the abdomen with almond oil scented with lavender tincture or cypress oil.

❦ An infusion of Saint Johnswort can help certain types of incontinence.

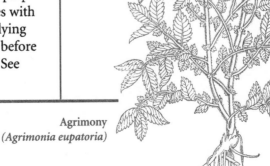

Agrimony
(Agrimonia eupatoria)

Liver Ailments, or Bilious Complaints

Recipe books generally offer remedies for the liver in the form of cures for "bilious complaints," or too much bile. Bile acts on the fats we consume, working like a detergent to break them up into digestible form. Occasionally, you may see remedies for a "bilious attack," however, which is usually a mislabeling of indigestion, or heartburn.

REMEDIES FOR THE LIVER

❦ Eat less meat; its digestion is hard on the liver.

❦ Eat tomatoes.

❦ Drink plenty of water.

❦ Avoid toxins in the environment as much as possible, including air pollution and workplace toxins (particularly substances found in dry-cleaning fluids, carpet adhesives, agricultural chemicals, lead paints and other paints, dyes, bleaches, and manufacturing of plastics and rubber).

❦ Exercise regularly enough to produce a sweat, which helps rid the body of toxins. Or, take regular saunas or steam baths.

❦ Increase your intake of vitamins C and E (a nontoxic antioxidant).

❦ Increase your consumption of fiber to help discharge the toxins you do ingest.

❦ Dandelion root, blessed thistle, and feverfew, in combination, make a good liver tonic.

❦ According to Andrew Weil, M.D., author of *Spontaneous Healing* (Alfred A. Knopf, 1995; Fawcett [paperback], 1996), "Anyone who is a heavy user of alcohol should take milk thistle regularly, as should patients using pharmaceutical drugs that are hard on the liver, including cancer patients undergoing chemotherapy." Bottled tinctures of milk thistle are found in health food stores.

Tomato
(*Lycopersicon lycopersicum*)

Dull the Appetite & Slim the Waist

In the 13th-century household of King Edward I of England, fennel and coriander seeds were stockpiled for use on the numerous fast days. Their effect was to dull the appetite rather than supply nutrition.

A recipe "for to make one slender" was published in the *Good Housewife's Jewel* (1585): "Take Fennel and seethe it in water, a very good quantity, and wring out the juice thereof, when it is sod, and drink it first and last, and it shall swage either him or her." The Greeks called fennel *marathon,* from *maraino,* meaning "to grow thin," and used it as a dietary broth to reduce unwieldiness.

The early English custom of afternoon tea may have begun in an effort to assuage hunger pangs and provide a calming beverage. Like various teas, especially sage tea, thyme was considered "good against the wambling and gripings of the bellie," according to the 17th-century herbalist John Gerard.

AIDS FOR DIETERS

❧ Add fennel to your diet to curb your appetite.

❧ Drink infusions of sage or thyme.

❧ Consider adding bulgur wheat to your diet. It's full of protein, niacin, and iron; low in sodium and fat; and a good source of fiber.

❧ Dieters benefit from adding more greens to their diets, such as collards, Swiss chard, beet greens, turnip greens, kale, and mustard greens. These also may lower the risks of cancer, high cholesterol, and diabetes. Add them to rice dishes or salads, or serve them steamed with feta cheese or slivered almonds.

❧ Some studies suggest that soup eaters lose weight more easily than those who shun soups. But make sure to avoid cream soups and soups that are high in meat fats.

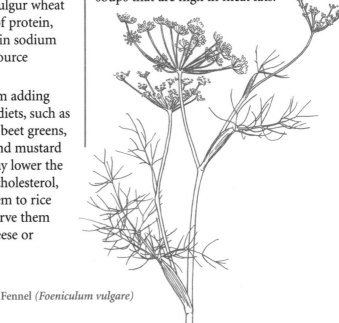

Fennel *(Foeniculum vulgare)*

❦ Dieters would do well to nearly eliminate meat and alcohol from their diets. (Pregnant and nursing women, convalescents, and those doing heavy manual labor need more protein than others, however, and might not want to eliminate meats.) They should increase their intake of fruits, grains, and vegetables and avoid refined foods.

❦ Certain types of drugs, such as birth control pills, cortisone pills, some migraine medications, and some mood stabilizers (such as lithium), can promote weight gain.

❦ Replace low-fiber foods with high-fiber equivalents to help make you feel full. For example, choose whole-wheat bread instead of white; beans, greens, and beets instead of summer squash or zucchini; or a baked potato instead of white rice.

❦ Kelp in your diet may help to reduce weight. It's rich in iodine and can help spark enzyme reactions.

❦ Don't skip any meals and eat more mini-meals to help shrink the stomach. Drink a glass of water with each mini-meal to help you feel full faster.

❦ Wear close-fitting clothes or a snug belt while dieting. A snug (but not tight) fit across the abdomen acts as a physical reminder to stop eating sooner.

❦ "For Extreme Fat: Use a total vegetable diet. I know one who was entirely cured of this by living a year thus: she breakfasted and supped on milk and water (with bread) and dined on turnips, carrots, or other roots, drinking water." (JW)

The Pain in Your Head

There are so many different kinds of headaches that one person's remedy may prove useless to someone else. Sinus involvement, food allergies, environmental conditions, caffeine withdrawal, drug reactions, eye problems, sleep deprivation, muscular tension, and stress are only a few of the things that might contribute to a headache. Migraines are a subject unto themselves, and much new research is being devoted to their cure. Listed below are remedies for various types of headaches. Keep in mind that determining the correct diagnosis of which type of headache you have can be the biggest headache of all.

REMEDIES FOR HEADACHES

❧ Some herbal teas to ease headaches include lavender (**Caution!** Keep dosages low if pregnant, or use externally), chamomile, elder flower, peppermint, feverfew (**Caution!** Avoid if pregnant), hops, skullcap, rosemary, and linden blossom. The oils of these same herbs, particularly the more aromatic ones (lavender, peppermint, and rosemary) are good for compresses for aromatherapy. Be sure to take time to inhale the steam from your tea!

❧ Studies done on feverfew leaves (eaten in a salad or sandwich) show promise for feverfew as a remedy for easing headaches and migraines. Feverfew also is a remedy for sinus conditions, premenstrual syndrome (PMS), and the headaches, cramps, and pains of difficult periods. Pregnant women should avoid it because it acts as a stimulant to the uterus. Anyone taking blood-thinning drugs also should avoid feverfew.

❧ Passionflower is used for migraines, nervous headaches, and stress.

❧ Lemon balm and rosemary are useful for menopausal symptoms, including headaches. Lemon balm is particularly useful for nervous disorders. Rosemary is considered rejuvenating, aiding clear thinking and increasing the flow of blood to the head. It is also useful for colds with fever and headache, as it helps to clear mucus and relieve air passages and lungs.

❧ Wood betony and skullcap are recommended for tension headaches. Both have mild sedative power. (**Caution!** Avoid high doses of wood betony if pregnant.)

❧ To help prevent a hangover headache, drink milk and eat fatty foods before indulging in alcohol. Choose white wine (or even better, a spritzer) over red, vodka over other hard liquors. Avoid very cheap wines, sweet wines, sherry, port, and sweetened liquors such as apricot brandy. Also avoid flavored, sweetened mixers, such as those used in strawberry daiquiris. Tonic water or club soda and citrus juices are fine.

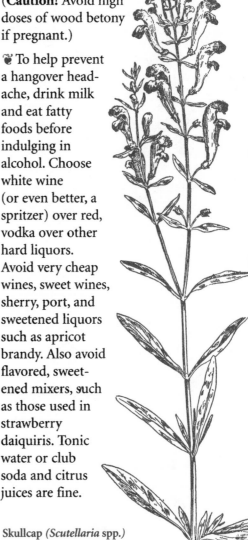

Skullcap (*Scutellaria* spp.)

🐞 For a hangover, try capsules of evening primrose, available at many health food stores.

🐞 Monosodium glutamate (MSG), often put in Chinese food, gives many people a headache. Request that it be left out of your food.

🐞 If you have headaches around your eyes, or if reading or other close work gives you a headache, get your eyes checked. You may need glasses or a new prescription.

🐞 Neck strain, tightness in the upper shoulders, squinting, and other forms of muscle tension can cause headaches. Try some simple yoga stretches for these areas. Wear sunglasses, especially if you are near the water or bright, snowy expanses such as ski slopes.

🐞 Caffeine withdrawal can cause a headache. If you have been a devoted coffee drinker and you stop cold turkey — say, because you're pregnant — you may get a headache. Sip a cola drink, green tea, or hot chocolate or replace some of the caffeine in another way until the headache eases.

🐞 Very cold foods, such as ice cream and iced drinks, can cause headaches.

> *When the head aches, all the members partake of the pains.*
>
> — MIGUEL DE CERVANTES (1547–1616)

🐞 Migraine headaches can be triggered by many things. Get to know which triggers you are most susceptible to and avoid them like the plague. Aside from certain foods, other possible migraine triggers are physical or mental exhaustion, including overwork and eyestrain; lack of exercise; smoking; air pollution; caffeine and withdrawal from caffeine; birth control pills and other drugs; menstrual fluctuations; hot or cold temperatures; and various digestive difficulties.

🐞 Even if you don't get migraines, you may get headaches from certain foods. For many people, salty foods are to blame. The headache may not start immediately but may come on an hour or more after you have ingested the foods.

🐞 For a sinus headache, apply a hot compress of plain water or an infusion of lavender, chamomile, or peppermint to the forehead. Lie down, breathing in the aroma. Replace the compress as necessary to keep it hot. (You may want to use two cloths, one always soaking in the bowl of hot infusion.) If you are using plain hot water, try wetting the compress, wringing it out, and microwaving it for a few seconds until hot.

❦ For a sinus headache, find the pressure points above the cheekbones or above your eyebrows and press lightly against them with your fingertips to clear the sinuses. When done correctly, you may hear a slight popping sound. You'll feel the release of tension in that area.

❦ Sinus headaches may respond to aromatic steam inhalations. Lavender, pine, eucalyptus, rosemary, and thyme are a few ingredients to try alone or in combination.

❦ Rub the temples with a small amount of tincture of lavender. The aroma, together with the brief massage, can relieve your headache.

❦ For a stress headache, lie down and close your eyes. Breathe deeply for a few minutes (for instruction, look up yoga breath exercises). Systematically erase from your mind any troubling thoughts.

❦ If you are getting headaches from hypertension, try adding garlic to your diet to lower your blood pressure.

❦ Sage tea and warm bricks to the feet are what Martha Ballard, midwife, prescribed in 1801 for a patient who had a pain in the head. When Ballard's daughter had "a severe pain in her head" (1795), the midwife applied a compress "feaver fue [feverfew] to her temples and Gave her a Clister [enema]. She Seemd Some Easier."

Heady Tea

Feverfew is especially good for migraine headaches. But if you are pregnant, make this tea with just the peppermint and rosemary.

2 parts peppermint leaves
2 parts feverfew leaves
1 part rosemary

Make an infusion, letting the herbs steep for at least 10 minutes.

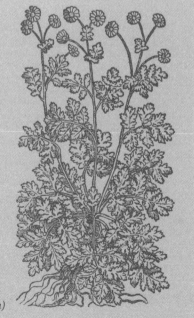

Feverfew *(Chrysanthemum parthenium)*

Chapter 6

Women's Complaints, Midwifery & the Moon

To my embarrassment I was born in bed with a lady.

— WILSON MIZNER (1876–1933)

Mugwort (*Artemisia vulgaris*)

Some say that the sun gives life, while the moon regulates it. Many cultures regard the sun as masculine and the moon as feminine. The tides, rain, reproduction and fertility, plant life, and even the life cycles of animals and humans all seem affected by the moon's gravitational pull. In herbal lore, the Greek moon goddess, Artemis (twin sister of Apollo, the sun god), reigns. You will see her name in several herbal remedies — most notably mugwort (*Artemisia vulgaris*) but also southernwood (*Artemisia abrotanum*) and wormwood (*Artemisia absinthium*) — all of which have links with childbirth and other gynecological conditions.

If the moon affects the tides, the moisture of the earth, and the well-being of all plants, isn't it plausible that it also affects our physical and mental well-being? Scientific studies over the years have tried to link the full moon with times of increased violence, suicide, mental disorders, fits and seizures, fertility or virility, and menstruation and birthing. Some small-scale studies have shown correlations between the full moon and increased police activity, "hot-line" calls, and hospital emergencies.

Not all of the moon's effects on health are considered negative. Just as many gardeners continue to plant by the moon, despite the lack of definitive corroboration, there are firm believers in performing medicine by the moon. The flow of blood especially has been suspected of responding to the gravitational tug of the moon.

Believers in the influence of the moon may consider dental care, elective surgery, and castration of animals unwise around the full moon because of the risk of increased bleeding. Similarly, Civil War doctors noted the tides, suspecting greater blood flow during a flood tide (high tide). A Florida physician, Dr. Edson Andrews, ran an informal study between 1956 and 1958 that pointed to excessive bleeding in operations done between the new and full (waxing) moon phases, with a peak at the full moon.

How does the moon affect you? Keep a moon chart that shows the waxing and waning phases of the moon handy, perhaps in your bathroom or bedroom. Notice how you feel during different phases of the moon. Do you sleep less well under a full moon? (See the section on insomnia in Chapter 7.) Are you bothered by bloating or water retention during certain phases? (Try the spring tonics in Chapter 4.) For women, note the menses in relation to the moon. Wristwatches with moon phases on the face can help make you more aware of the moon. Keep a diary of the phases and note how you feel. Over a few months, you may notice some correlations.

THE MOON, THE TIDE & YOU

❧ Moon lore says to fill cavities during a waning moon. Extract teeth during the early waxing period.

❧ Likewise, surgery is best performed during the early waxing period, when wounds heal faster. However, if the surgery is for removal of warts, calluses, or other unwanted growths, it's best to use the waning period and when the signs are "in the feet," such as in Capricorn or Pisces.

❧ Don't commence weaning (or, ideally, birthing) when the moon is waning.

❧ An early Roman custom was for women to wear silver crescent moons on their shoes to be sure of bearing healthy children.

❧ Moon lore suggests that you should cut your hair when the moon is in the daily zodiac signs of Pisces, Cancer, or Scorpio (watery signs) if you want it to grow back faster. An increasing moon phase is best. For slower growth, cut your hair during Leo, Virgo, or Gemini and when the

∽∘∼

[The moon] replenishes the earth; when she approaches it, she fills all bodies, while, when she recedes, she empties them.

— PLINY THE ELDER (A.D. 23–79)

∽∘∼

moon is on the wane.

❧ If you live near the ocean, you may begin to notice the ebb and flow of the tides, which are connected to the moon. Do you find the sound of the ocean relaxing? Use it to unwind when you are stressed.

❧ Walt Whitman noted the effects of tides and moon phases when he visited Civil War hospitals. He remarked that drugs seemed more effective and deaths gentler when they came with the ebb or flood tides (low or high tides).

❧ To be born at flood tide was considered lucky. In sickness, the ebb tide was a time of weakness and extra caution, especially for old salts. If a patient survived the ebb, he might improve in strength with the flood. The full moon carried similar lore; it was con-sidered a time of births but also of increased bleeding and greater susceptibility to sickness.

❧ An evening walk in the moon-light or an evening sail under a full moon can be particularly relaxing.

Women's Complaints

Many of the remedies for women's complaints include the worts, such as motherwort and birthwort, and other herbs that name women in some form. For example, you'll frequently see references to lady's-mantle, lady's slipper (*American valerian*), mother's-heart (shepherd's purse), squawroot (black cohosh), and the like. Others give hints about their usage in their Latin names. Damiana, for instance, sometimes includes *aphrodisiaca* as part of its Latin name, indicating its stimulating action on the reproductive system. Since many early herbalists were women, often working as midwives, there's no scarcity of remedies for gynecological problems.

THE MENSES

Since a woman's period has a cycle that resembles that of the moon, it is not surprising that *menstruation* derives from "moon change." In French, it is *le moment de la lune*. Some women can predict the onset of their periods according to the changes of the moon.

❦ A diet to aid the body during menstruation should contain plenty of vitamin B$_6$ (sunflower seeds, lentils, lima beans, pinto beans, black-eyed peas, rice bran, broccoli, asparagus).

❦ Ginger, in hot ginger tea or mixed with milk, is an old remedy for the pain associated with menstruation.

❦ An infusion of lady's-mantle can be used for regulating the menses and helping to prevent premenstrual syndrome (PMS). A few drops of wood betony or mugwort tincture can be added to the infusion. (**Caution!** Avoid if pregnant.)

❦ PMS sufferers may want to avoid alcohol, caffeine, sugar, chocolate, cola, and tobacco. Blood sugar balance may be critical to keeping yourself on an even keel. Don't skip meals or indulge sugar cravings. Consider taking a multivitamin and be sure it contains vitamin B$_6$, vitamin E, and zinc.

❦ Peppermint and vervain (verbena), in decocted form, ease PMS.

❦ According to some Native Americans, yarrow tea eases and shortens heavy periods.

❦ Shepherd's purse, also called mother's-heart, in an infusion of its aerial parts, eases heavy periods. Goldenseal tincture can be added.

❦ The spring tonic herbs (see Chapter 4), such as burdock root, dandelion, and corn silk, can be helpful in minimizing fluid retention, which can cause cramps or a bloated feeling during the menses.

❦ A decoction of rhubarb roots can be taken for menstrual cramps. (**Caution!** Avoid if pregnant; rhubarb acts as a purgative.)

❦ Decocted basil, in a strong tea, can ease the pain and cramps of heavy periods.

❦ Women with heavy periods should take extra care to avoid anemia by increasing their intake of iron-rich foods and foods with vitamin C, which helps in iron absorption.

❦ Black currant, in jellies, jams, teas, syrups, and other forms, is often helpful in relieving menstrual difficulties.

❦ For some women, a hot-water bottle or heating pad relieves menstrual cramps.

❦ Some women soak their feet in a mustard bath to bring on the menses or to ease cramps.

❦ Medieval and Renaissance herbalists used parsley, a uterine stimulant, to bring on the menses.

❦ Raspberries, red or black, and raspberry teas are reputed to be relaxing to the uterus and may be helpful for menstrual cramps.

❦ Squawroot, also called black cohosh, black snakeroot, and rattlesnake root, is a Native American remedy for painful periods. (**Caution!** Too high a dose may cause dizziness. Avoid if pregnant.)

❦ Other herbs reputed to ease menstrual cramps include allspice, angelica, bee balm, lemon balm, black haw, chamomile, feverfew, rosemary, thyme, and valerian.

❦ Celery seed is reputed to ease water retention.

❦ Try active exercise, such as a brisk walk, for relief of cramps. It's often more effective than curling up in bed because it stimulates circulation. Yoga stretches can be helpful as well.

Cramp Relievers

Here are two teas to ease menstrual cramps.

Saint Johnswort & Raspberry Tea
Infuse equal parts Saint Johnswort leaves and raspberry leaves in boiling water for 10 minutes.

Cinnamon Tea
Combine ½ teaspoon ground cinnamon and 1 cup boiling water.

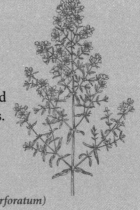

Saint Johnswort *(Hypericum perforatum)*

YEAST INFECTIONS

Not all vaginal inflammations are yeast infections. When in doubt or if symptoms persist, consult your medical practitioner.

❦ Make an infusion of pot marigold petals and use as a douche.

❦ Consume raw garlic in your daily diet to prevent and treat yeast infections.

❦ Consume yogurt with active cultures to help prevent yeast infections. Plain yogurt also can be used as a topical cleanser, applied in the shower and rinsed away after a few minutes. It is cooling and helps relieve itching and restore proper balance.

❦ Goldenseal tincture, diluted with water, can be used as a douche for yeast infections, vaginitis, or itching.

❦ A douche of infused red clover helps eliminate vaginal itching. A douche of infused plantain leaves does the same. If you have the seeds, soak them in a small amount of boiling water. They will form a gel, which can be very soothing to any areas of irritation on the more external parts.

❦ A douche of apple cider vinegar, much diluted with warm water, helps prevent or relieve vaginal itching. Because of its acidity, do not use too frequently or where there is already redness or irritation.

❦ Drink cranberry juice. (Seek organic sources.)

❦ Reduce your sugar intake.

❦ Avoid using tampons, which can spread a yeast infection.

❦ Antibiotics, hormone replacement therapy, and birth control pills can increase your susceptibility to yeast infections. If you must continue their use and are having trouble with yeast infections, consult your medical practitioner about possible substitutes. Meanwhile, use the preceding suggestions to help build up your resistance. Herbal teas, such as one made with the roots of purple coneflower, also may be helpful in building up your immune system.

❦ Drink cinnamon tea (about ½ teaspoon ground cinnamon in 1 cup boiling water) or add a cinnamon stick to your regular tea or hot cider.

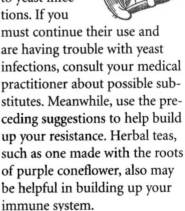

Marigold
(Calendula
officinalis)

FERTILITY

❦ If you are trying to get pregnant, look for herbs that stimulate the reproductive system (for example, peppermint and marigold flowers). Others, such as ginseng, false unicorn root, and blue cohosh, help regulate hormones.

❦ Various seaweeds (kelp), high in minerals, are suggested to promote fertility.

❦ The cleansing tonics (see Chapter 4) can be very helpful for women who want to become pregnant. Some of these tonics also provide vitamin C, which is recommended to enhance fertility and help absorb much-needed iron. Some recent studies suggest that a sufficient level of vitamin C, even before conception, can help prevent certain birth defects. Red clover, stinging nettles, and burdock root are a few of the recommended potherbs. Red clover simulates estrogen compounds, which can be helpful as well.

❦ "Mrs. Lydia E. Pinkham's Vegetable Compound" (label patented in 1876) was prescribed for "Prolapsis Uteri, or falling of the Womb, and all Female Weaknesses, including Leucorrhea [vaginal discharge], painful menstruation, inflammation, and ulceration of the womb, irregularities, floodings, etc."

The compound contained false unicorn root, liferoot, black cohosh, pleurisy root, and fenugreek seeds, macerated and bottled in a solution of about 19 percent alcohol.

❦ A study by the Oxford (England) Family Planning Association, run over the course of 5 years with 4,000 women, showed that women who smoked as many as 16 cigarettes a day conceived only half as often as nonsmokers. Zinc absorption, decreased by smoking, seemed to be the link. Birth control pills and high-fiber diets also decrease zinc absorption. Men and women seeking to increase their zinc absorption should eat leafy green vegetables, fish, nuts, wheat germ, and meats, with an emphasis on organic sources.

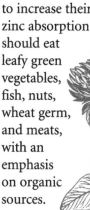

Red clover
(*Trifolium pratense*)

MENOPAUSE

Like the beginning of menstruation, menopause — literally, the last period — is a time of change for a woman, both physically and emotionally. In a society with, at best, mixed messages about aging, it's easy for a woman to feel that diminishing value is being given her place in the world. Even for the most confident women, saying good-bye to the reproductive years can bring sadness. But menopause also can be freeing. Some women come into their own as they escape societal expectations of them primarily as wives and mothers.

❦ Motherwort, to be avoided during pregnancy, is useful in menopause as a mild sedative and uterine tonic. Make an infusion of the leaves and flowers. A few drops of a tincture of sage, mugwort, lavender, wood betony, or lady's-mantle may be added as well.

❦ Saint Johnswort, in an infusion of its aerial parts or as a tincture added to other teas, can be taken for menopausal symptoms, including anxiety, irritability, insomnia, depression, and tension.

❦ The chaste berry, available from health food stores in tincture form, can be helpful to restore hormonal balance and ease the symptoms of menopause. Avoid high doses, which can cause a prickly sensation on the skin.

❦ An infusion of basil can be effective for minimizing the night sweats of menopause.

❦ Ginseng tea is often recommended for menopause, both for its B vitamins and minerals and for its reputation as a rejuvenator and restorer of sexual libido.

❦ Hot flashes may respond to a tea of sage and mugwort, in equal parts. The same works for night sweats. Some people recommend sage tea alone, calling sage "the night-sweat remedy."

❦ Midwife Martha Ballard, in 1805 at the age of 80, when she was "not So wel as I could wish," took "a beer made of hops and Balm Gilliad." Although she was certainly well past menopause, it is worth noting that hops contain estrogenic substances, while the balm of Gilead (from a North American poplar tree) contains salicin, giving it properties similar to those of aspirin.

❦ Calendula, hops, ginseng, sage, and wild yam exhibit an estrogenic action that can be helpful during menopause. Rhubarb, tofu, miso, oats, alfalfa, and celery also contain estrogen-simulating substances.

HYSTERECTOMY

Whole books have been written on the subject of hysterectomies. If your medical practitioner has not given you a clear idea of what to expect, educate yourself on the subject. If possible, talk with several women who've undergone the operation. Depression, melancholy, early menopause, and other physical and emotional disorders are often associated with this procedure. In early India, the Ayurveda healers associated the uterus with the root chakra (according to yoga philosophy, one of the seven centers of spiritual energy in the human body). Removal of the uterus, they believed, might prompt an imbalance leading to a lack of concentration, restlessness, and an unsettled state. In addition to the following remedies, those suggested for menopause (see page 87) are recommended for early menopause brought on by hysterectomy.

🌱 Basil leaves, consumed in the daily diet through salads or pesto, can act as an antidepressant and prevent melancholy.

🌱 Wood betony, in an infusion of its aerial parts, can be taken as both a mild sedative and a stimulant to the circulation in the head, for better concentration and focus.

🌱 Massage the temples with lavender oil to ease anxiety.

🌱 For melancholy or depression, drink rosemary tea by itself or combined with skullcap or vervain.

🌱 Women who have had a total hysterectomy are at greater risk of developing osteoporosis. They should take added precautions against this (see below).

OSTEOPOROSIS

For many women, menopause also means loss of bone density, because with the sharp decrease in estrogen at menopause comes a parallel increase in the need for calcium — a need we tend to overlook. Even before menopause, it's wise to be aware of your calcium intake.

🌱 For women over 35 who hope to reduce their risk of osteoporosis, exercise is key to maintaining good bone strength and density. Swimming, because it is not "weight bearing" (the water takes your weight), is not a good choice. Walking, running, dancing, and aerobics are better alternatives.

🌱 Choose foods from local and organic sources so that you minimize the risk of food additives or pesticides that might contaminate them. Foods from organic farms also may have higher vitamin and mineral content than produce from intensively farmed areas with more depleted soils.

🌿 Do not assume that drinking an extra glass of milk (or adding other dairy products) will meet your calcium needs. It's more complicated than that. For proper calcium absorption, you need adequate (but not immoderate) amounts of vitamin D. Get out the sun, which helps your body make vitamin D. If you are taking a daily multivitamin, check the balance of these ingredients. If you take supplements only, include calcium, vitamin D, and magnesium.

🌿 Sources of calcium include milk, greens, dried fruits, bony fish, enriched cereals, seeds, and nuts.

🌿 Vitamin D is available from milk, eggs, fatty fish, and fish oils.

🌿 Magnesium is available from hard water, eggs, milk, greens, seafood, and many seeds and nuts.

🌿 Be aware of your phosphorus intake, shooting for roughly equal amounts of calcium and phosphorus. Cottage cheese has a good balance of calcium and phosphorus.

🌿 Pasta is a good source of phosphorus, as are seeds, nuts, fish, grains, and eggs. Some studies link a high-meat, high-dairy diet with osteoporosis. Although meats and dairy foods are high in phosphorus, they offer a poor overall balance of vitamins and minerals.

🌿 Low-fat yogurt, sardines, most greens (collards, spinach, kale, turnip greens, and so on), salmon, oysters, bean burritos, baked beans, soybeans, broccoli, and scallops are all sources of calcium. However, some foods, such as spinach and rhubarb, also reduce your absorption of minerals, so you'll want to use them in moderation and, if possible, eat them separately from other sources of minerals. Eating a wide variety of foods is your best bet. (**Caution!** Keep in mind that calcium-rich foods may contribute to kidney stones and may reduce the effectiveness of tetracycline [an antibiotic]. If you have trouble with either of these, consult a medical practitioner before changing your calcium intake.)

🌿 Various seaweeds (kelp), high in minerals, help prevent osteoporosis.

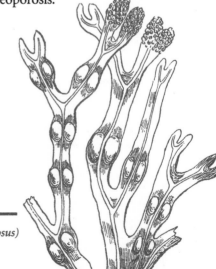

Kelp (*Fucus vesiculosus*)

The Midwife's Domain

The list of herbs in midwife Martha Ballard's (1735–1812) garden gives us some idea of her remedies. Besides the turnips, parsnips, peppers, currants, quince, and rhubarb — which might be either supper or remedy — herbs included anise, burnet, catnip, chamomile, coriander, feverfew, flax, garlic, hops, hyssop, mandrake, marigolds, mints, mustard, parsley, peppergrass, rue, saffron, sage, savory, spearmint, tansy, and numerous others. Ballard speaks frequently of her "clysters" (enemas, often of chamomile), plasters, poultices, "pukes" (emetics), and salves. But of all her remedies, the herbal teas are by far the most common, prescribed for everything from "stomach colics" to "sore Travel" (travail, or labor).

MORNING SICKNESS

❦ Many women find that some simple cracker is all they need to get them through the early morning sickness of pregnancy. This nausea is misnamed, coming as it does at any hour of the day. However, if you considered the 40 weeks or so of a full-term pregnancy as a day, then you could say the nausea comes in the "morning" portion; it's generally gone by the second trimester.

❦ Like other forms of nausea, morning sickness responds well to ginger. Sip ginger tea, eat ginger cookies (see the recipe on page 66), or take ground ginger in capsule form. Do not overdo it —

moderation in all things, especially in early pregnancy, should always be your rule of thumb.

❦ Other teas that can alleviate morning sickness include chamomile, rosemary, lavender, fennel, basil, peppermint, skullcap, and lemon balm. It's better to alternate several varieties than to rely on just one.

❦ Avoid very strong smells that may upset a squeamish stomach.

❦ Eliminating dairy or wheat products from the diet for a short time may help alleviate morning sickness.

❦ Try black haw to relieve morning sickness.

❦ Take slippery elm jelly (see the recipe on page 26) when you feel the nausea coming on.

Black haw (*Viburnum prunifolium*)

MISCARRIAGE

Though difficult to do, it's wise to keep in mind that many miscarriages are nature's way of ending a pregnancy where the prognosis was not good. If this is the case, no remedy can change that, nor would you want it to. Other factors, including general health and nutrition, proper rest, hormonal balance, and the health of both partners' reproductive systems, all play a part. The remedies listed below are just a few to consider in the overall scheme of things.

🍃 If you smoke, stop!

🍃 Do not drink alcoholic beverages while pregnant.

🍃 It's critical to avoid the cat's litter box and feces because of the risk of toxoplasmosis.

🍃 Avoid raw meats, which also can cause toxoplasmosis. If you must handle them, use rubber gloves and wash well afterward. Be sure all meat is well cooked before you eat it.

🍃 Use moderation in all things, including foods, herbs, drinks, exercise, sex, and other exertions. Listen to what your body is telling you. If you're tired, get more sleep.

🍃 Motherwort (the aerial parts) has a reputation for preventing miscarriage, but it should be noted that it is a gentle uterine stimulant as well as an antispasmodic and relaxant. More often, it is used for delayed periods (to bring them on) and toward the end of a full-term pregnancy to tone the uterus and prepare for birth. Some use it to ease or prevent false labor pains.

🍃 Reduce or eliminate your intake of caffeine in coffee, tea, cola, chocolate, and other foods.

🍃 False unicorn root is an ovarian and uterine tonic reputed to help prevent miscarriage. It is also used for painful periods and is often combined (for either purpose) with cramp bark. Both are prepared through decoction.

🍃 In general, avoid the herbs used to bring on the menses, which may be uterine stimulants that could cause untimely contractions. Parsley, for example, while probably harmless in small doses, is sometimes present in large quantities in certain pesto recipes and in tabbouleh. Avoid rhubarb, rue, goldenseal, mugwort, tansy, nutmeg, calendula, feverfew, and sage. Don't make yourself crazy about it, however; a sprinkling of nutmeg in an apple pie won't hurt you!

🍃 Black haw is a mild sedative and antispasmodic that is sometimes recommended to prevent miscarriage.

Cramp bark (*Viburnum opulus*)

CHILDBIRTH

Many modern-day midwives have extensive knowledge of soothing and healing herbs, tonics, teas, salves, and massage oils for both pregnancy and birthing. In the early stages of your pregnancy, talk with other women and various health practitioners to find out what resources are available in your area. Some women put together a kit of remedies and relaxation aids for their pregnancy and delivery. This kit can help a partner to become more actively involved in assisting during labor and birthing as well.

❧ A cup of raspberry leaf tea helps tone the uterus before birth. Take one cup (some herbalists recommend up to three cups) a day in the last weeks of pregnancy. Some people believe that it helps shorten the duration of labor.

❧ There may be some truth to the belief that women go into an energetic spurt of "nesting" (washing floors, painting the nursery, doing spring cleaning) just before labor commences. Avoid this urge so that you won't be exhausted when labor begins. If you must paint the nursery, ventilate the room well and wear a charcoal-filtered face mask to avoid breathing in the fumes.

❧ The last days before delivery can be physically stressful, making you more susceptible to colds and flu. Take added precautions to enhance your immune system through rest, proper diet, and exercise. You may need extra care in regulating your diet to avoid constipation. If you know some yoga, meditation, or massage tech-niques, use them now. If you don't, consider learning some.

❧ Add small amounts of cinna-mon, nutmeg, cloves, sage, and ginger to your cooking in the last few weeks of your pregnancy to help tone your reproductive organs for an easier delivery. Keep quantities in moderation, using no more than ordinary recipes would call for.

❧ Lavender tea during birthing, or a soothing massage with laven-der oil diluted in sweet olive or almond oil, may help prevent exhaustion. (**Caution!** Do not use before labor; lavender is a uterine stimulant.)

❧ To help ease "back labor" or **backaches during transition** (advanced stage of labor), use massage oils made of sweet olive and/or almond oil with a tincture of sage, rose, lavender, or chamomile.

❧ To ease the exhaustion of a long labor, use massage oils for foot massage. Some people find that an automatic vibrator is particularly useful for this purpose. It can be used for the lower back as well.

❧ A teaspoon of the dried leaves and flowers of wood betony, taken in a weak infusion (at least a cup of water), can ease labor. It is a mild sedative but also a uterine stimulant.

❧ Many birthing centers in progressive hospitals are adding whirlpool baths to their facilities. At certain times in early labor and during the birthing process, the warm water and gentle massage can help women relax through the contractions. Aromatic bath ingredients such as bergamot, chamomile, hops, lavender, mint, oat straw, rosemary, sage, thyme, and valerian can be added, in small cheesecloth bags or in tea bags, for their relaxing effects. For pregnant women with itchy skin, yellow dock or plantain added to the bath will bring relief. (See Chapter 7 for more on aromatic remedies.)

To Ease Labor & Prevent Afterpains

To Ease Labor
½ pound figs
½ pound raisins
4 ounces licorice root, scraped and sliced
1 teaspoon anise seed, bruised
2 quarts spring water

Boil the figs, raisins, licorice, and anise seed in the water until the liquid is reduced by one-half. Strain. Drink 4 ounces of it morning and evening for six weeks before the baby's due date.

To Prevent Afterpains
½ ounce ground nutmeg
2 egg whites
1 ounce ground cinnamon

Mix together the nutmeg and cinnamon. Combine with the egg whites and beat the mixture together in a small bowl. "Take every morning in bed as much as will lie on the point of a knife, and so at night."

Adapted from *The Compleat Housewife: or, Accomplish'd Gentlewoman's Companion* by E. Smith (1753).

Nutmeg (*Myristica fragrans*)

THE POSTPARTUM PERIOD

❦ An infusion of motherwort leaves (see page 129) can be taken as a tea during labor or after the birthing to help restore the uterus and minimize postpartum bleeding. Motherwort is both a relaxant and a uterine stimulant.

❦ Motherwort and basil, combined in an infused tea, are recommended immediately after birthing to help ensure that the placenta separates properly and is not retained.

❦ False unicorn root makes a soothing and rejuvenating tea after the birth of a child. Drink it as a tonic up to three times a day.

❦ Drink raspberry leaf tea to help bring the uterus back into condition after childbirth.

❦ A tea of Saint Johnswort and calendula, mixed in equal parts, is both healing and a good preventive against depression or "postpartum blues."

❦ Other teas useful against postpartum depression include rosemary, skullcap, lemon balm, and wild oat.

❦ Essential oils for massage that help counteract postpartum blues include bergamot, clary sage, rose, and angelica.

❦ For hemorrhoids, make an infusion of the bark of the maidenhair tree (*Ginkgo biloba*) and use as a wash.

❦ Tonic herbs (see Chapter 4), such as burdock root, stinging nettles, and dandelion, help maintain your levels of iron and calcium during the natural bleeding that follows childbirth. They also assist in detoxifying your system and restoring hormonal balance.

❦ For women who have had an episiotomy, mild herbal washes of infused calendula, chamomile, comfrey, plantain, Saint Johnswort, or witch hazel, diluted with warm water, promote healing. Once the area is somewhat healed, salves such as calendula or plantain can be applied directly to the area, but the washes are best early on. (See Chapter 7 for other aromatic baths.)

❦ Sitz baths with infusions of goldenseal root, comfrey leaves, plantain, yarrow, or calendula can help heal postpartum swelling, torn perineal tissue, or an episiotomy.

❦ Martha Ballard, in 1790, gave Mrs. Cragg (who had been four days in labor and finally delivered a first-born daughter) a relaxing "Bath of Tansey, mugwort, Cammomile & Hysop, which gave mrs Cragg great relief."

❦ Breast-feeding helps the uterus contract after childbirth and return to its normal position and muscle tone.

BREAST CARE & BREAST-FEEDING

❦ The petals of pot marigold are available in various cream and salve forms at most health food stores. Apply to cracked or sore nipples immediately after breast-feeding. Wipe off before the next feeding.

❦ If you or your baby objects to the pot marigold, with its distinctive, rather bitter smell, you can make a breast cream from honey and almond oil. Use as often as needed. Apply after breast-feeding.

❦ A poultice of mashed cabbage leaves or mashed turnips may help ease mastitis. If you haven't time to lie down with the poultice, soak a cabbage leaf in very warm water until it is soft, then apply it to the breast between your skin and your bra. Leave it in place for 15 minutes or longer. Apply fresh leaves as necessary. Your baby may dislike the taste, so wipe the breast clean before nursing.

❦ More frequent feedings, even if of short duration, will help increase the flow of breast milk.

❦ Some of the herbs considered helpful in increasing the flow of milk are fennel, milk thistle, fenugreek, dill, raspberry leaves, blessed thistle, stinging nettles, false unicorn root, and cinnamon. Add any or all to your daily diet. Avoid if you are weaning.

❦ To Increase Milk: "Drink a pint of water before going to bed. Or, drink largely of pottage [thick soup] made with lentils." (JW)

❦ To Increase Milk in Nurses: "Make gruel with lentils, and let the party drink freely of it; or else boil them in posset-drink, which they like best." (ES)

❦ Some women say that a bottle of stout beer at the end of the day helps relax them and maintain their milk supply. Stouts often contribute some iron, but be mindful of the alcohol content. If you do choose this remedy, you might do well to drink your stout just after breast-feeding so that the alcohol in your system has time to dissipate before the next feeding.

❦ To reduce breast milk for weaning, drink sage or peppermint tea. Avoid these if you are continuing to breast-feed.

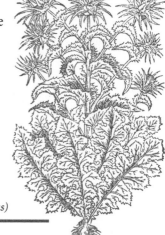

Milk thistle
(*Carduus marianus*)

Chapter 7

Aromatics to Calm & Revive

As aromatic plants bestow
No spicy fragrance while they grow;
But crush'd or trodden to the ground,
Diffuse their balmy sweets around.

— OLIVER GOLDSMITH (1728–1774)

Lavender
(*Lavendula officinalis*)

A romatic remedies take many forms. They are probably among our most ancient remedies, but they also have the strongest foothold in contemporary usage. Old herbals prescribed the calming scents of thyme and sage leaf teas for nightmares or "night-ghosts," and bald men were told to wash their heads with sage tea to grow hair. Lemony bee balm tea was prescribed for longevity, licorice-like fennel for better eyesight, lady's-mantle (the "alchemist's herb") for acne and female troubles, and lovage as a deodorant. Rosemary tea is reviving, rather than sedative, and also reputed to aid memory and ease migraines. Many of the most fragrant herbs were the ones found along the outside borders of early medicinal gardens, probably for their ability to ward off pests.

Herbal shampoos and hair rinses were once used to induce sleep as well as cleanse the hair. Chamomile leaves and flowers and decocted dill seed were both sprinkled on the hair or pillow to cure insomnia. Dill, from the Saxon word meaning "to lull," also would "hinder witches from their will." Its fragrance lulled cranky or colicky babies to sleep. Decocted sassafras bark was considered a more powerful hair rinse, reputed to kill head lice. Fennel leaves were sometimes stuffed in bedroom keyholes to ward off nightmares. Ozark sleeping aids included putting jimsonweed in the shoes, then setting the shoes under the bed. The same herb was used in tea to treat nervous ailments.

In blending teas or shampoos or in making sleep pillows, let your nose be your guide. Just as with flowers or perfumes, what constitutes a blissful scent to one may be repugnant to another.

Before experimenting with aromatics for the bath or complexion, perform a 24-hour skin test. Take a tiny amount of the herb to be used, whether fresh or dried, and pulverize it with a mortar and pestle. If it's dried, add a few drops of water to moisten it. Dab the paste on the inside of your forearm, cover with a bandage, and let it sit for 24 hours. Then check for any sign of skin irritation or reaction — redness, blistering, itching, or swelling. If you're clear, it should be safe to use externally.

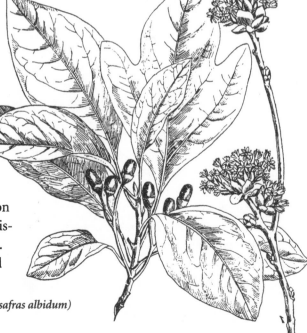

Sassafras (*Sassafras albidum*)

FOR THE BATH

❦ Dried lavender flowers, added to the bath, offer a fragrant soak and mild astringent cleansing. Lavender is antibacterial as well. This is a good choice for young children and colicky babies.

❦ Add the lemony bee balm leaves, fresh or dried in a cheesecloth bag or tea bag, to your bath to soothe frayed nerves, relieve cramps, and aid sleep.

❦ Sprigs of rosemary in the bath offer a piny fragrance. (You also could add pine needles, reputed to relieve nervous tension, if that's the scent you crave.) Rosemary is considered invigorating and also is good for aches and pains and for a tired complexion. Some people consider its fragrance an aphrodisiac. Others find it too strong and get headaches from it. Eucalyptus or bay leaves can be used for the same effect.

❦ Full baths, footbaths, or compresses using freshly grated gingerroot can help break a fever, induce sweating, improve circulation to sore joints, or ease tired feet. For a footbath, sit on a chair over the bath, then wrap a warm blanket around yourself so that it envelops the steaming bath as well.

❦ In the past, hot footbaths, given their heat by mustard or lye, were used to relieve headaches.

❦ Some Native Americans took sponge baths with decocted verbena leaves to combat nervousness. You might try this along with verbena tea for added effectiveness.

❦ Native Americans also took hot sage baths for shaky, cramping, or weakened legs. Or a sage poultice was applied directly to the legs.

❦ Calendula, comfrey, and chamomile can be used separately or together for an astringent bath that is especially helpful for those with oily or blemished skin. They also can be infused and mixed with a decoction of distilled water and witch hazel bark to make a facial cleanser. Calendula and chamomile are particularly useful for young children and babies.

❦ For a highly curative chamomile bath, combine 1 pound chamomile flowers and 20 gallons hot water. This is good for skin irritations, inflammations such as bedsores, and hemorrhoids.

❦ Take a cup of chamomile tea, made with two tea bags, into the bath with you. Let the infusion steep briefly, then lift the tea bags out and allow them to cool slightly. Place one over each eyelid to ease puffiness or irritation and aid relaxation. When they cool too much, put them back in the hot tea water, then dip them out again and reapply.

❦ Elder flowers steeped in hot water make a gently cleansing bath with only a slight floral scent. They also are considered sleep inducing and relaxing to the nerves.

❧ For rough skin, take a bath in comfrey, reputed to be rejuvenating to the skin. For chapped hands, use a salve of comfrey or mix an infusion of comfrey with some glycerin or rose water. (**Caution!** Not for internal use.)

❧ Add milk, liquid or powdered, to the bath to counteract hard water and smooth the skin. (Cleopatra used camel's milk.) Bath salts, oils, or herbs also can be added.

Relaxing Herbal Bath Tea Bags

A relaxing herbal bath can be as simple as adding a few commercial tea bags to the water. Some people like to steep the bags in boiling water first, then add them to the bath. Others use very hot tap water, add the tea bags, and get in when the water has cooled to a comfortable temperature. To make your own bath teas, try this recipe, experimenting with other ingredients of your choice.

Make a cheesecloth bag by sewing a folded packet, or simply use a twist tie or bit of string to close the bag.

½ cup grated fresh gingerroot

2 tablespoons one or more of the following dried (unless otherwise indicated) herbs:

lemon verbena	**lemon balm**
rosemary sprigs (fresh or dried)	**sweet marjoram**
any of the mints (fresh or dried)	**grated goldenseal root**
chamomile	**plantain leaves**
lavender	

Combine the gingerroot and the herbs. Insert the ingredients in the bag and add it to your bath.

Bath tea bags should be used only once. If you make them as gifts, be sure to include a label identifying the herbs you have used so that the recipient can beware of any skin sensitivities.

Rosemary *(Rosmarinus officinalis)*

FOR THE COMPLEXION

❧ Drink plenty of water, around eight glasses a day, either plain or in noncaffeinated teas or carbonated waters (not colas). Increase your water consumption in cold and/or dry climates or when subjected to the drying heat of wood stoves, furnaces, or car heaters or to other low-humidity conditions, such as on airplanes.

❧ Add brewer's yeast to your daily diet.

❧ Stay out of the hot sun! Tanning and sunburns dry out your skin.

❧ Avoid detergent-type soaps with dyes and other additives.

❧ Aftershave: Rosemary and sage, used separately, are frequent choices. Both are astringent and stimulating to the skin. For oily skin or for sunburns, sage is the better choice. Either one can be combed into your hair or beard as well.

❧ To help prevent and reduce wrinkles, use hops in skin creams, oils, or salves to soften the skin. Apply with light, upward massage strokes or a patting motion rather than rubbing or dragging against the skin.

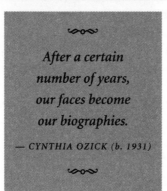

After a certain number of years, our faces become our biographies.

— CYNTHIA OZICK (b. 1931)

❧ For a quick skin toner, use equal parts white or apple cider vinegar and water. Lemon juice may be substituted for the vinegar.

❧ Powdered rose hips, made into a paste, are reputed to remove freckles and liver spots (age spots).

❧ Lovage is another herb reputed to remove freckles and clear up redness in the face. It has antibiotic properties.

❧ Lip Salve: "Take a quarter of a pound of alkanet root [henna] bruised, and half a quarter of a pound of fresh butter, as much bees-wax, and a pint of claret; boil all these together a pretty while; then strain it, and let it stand till it is cold; then take the wax off the top, and melt it again, and pour it clear from the dregs into your gallipots or boxes: use it when and as often as you please." (ES)

❧ "Oyle of Camomile: Take oyle a pint and a halfe, and 3 ounces of camomile flowers dried one day after they be gathered. Then put the oyle and the flowers in a glasse and stop the mouth close and set it into the Sun by the space of 40 days." (*The Good Housewife's Handbook*, 1588)

❦ For Pimples: "Take wheat-flour mingled with honey and vinegar, and lay on the pimples going to bed." (ES)

❦ Make a paste of baking soda and water and apply directly to facial blemishes. Let sit until dry, then rinse.

❦ For a facial steam, combine thyme, lavender, and chamomile in a bowl of steaming water. Make a tent over your head with a towel and bathe your face in the vapors for five to ten minutes to refresh the skin.

❦ Some oils considered helpful for preventing wrinkles include borage seed, clary sage, fennel, lavender, carrot, yarrow, frankincense, myrrh, lemon, hyssop, oregano, orange, vervain (verbena), rosemary, evening primrose, lime, and violet leaf.

❦ For oily skin or blackheads, make an infusion of yarrow with milk instead of water, apply to the skin, let dry, and rinse.

❦ For acne, rub the affected area with a clove of garlic (antibacterial and antifungal).

❦ Decoct cabbage leaves and strain, using the water as an anti-inflammatory acne wash. For greater cleansing and astringent action, combine with witch hazel.

❦ Take 1 cup elder flowers, cover with 1 pint boiling water, and let steep, covered, for 24 hours. Strain and use as is for a facial wash, or mix with 1 tablespoon lemon juice for a facial astringent.

❦ If your face is very dry, massage it with honey. As an occasional cleanser, add oats to the honey and use as a facial scrub. A small amount of chamomile, mint, or parsley could be added for a more fragrant, refreshing mask. Rinse with warm water.

Applesauce Face Mask

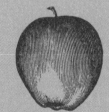

Apple (*Pyrus malus*)

This is especially good for oily skin.

- 1 apple, quartered
- 1 teaspoon lemon juice
- 1 teaspoon dried herb (parsley, sage, rosemary, lavender, peppermint, spearmint, chamomile, calendula, or other herb of your choice)

Cook the apple in water until it can be mashed. Mash the pulp and strain, discarding the solids. Add the lemon juice and herb and mix well. Apply to the face as a mask. Leave on for 5 minutes, then rinse with warm water and apply a moisturizer.

❦ Olive oil, almond oil, or vitamin E oil can be used to treat very dry skin before a shower. Apply all over and let sit while the shower is heating up and the steam permeates the room. Then enter the shower and rinse off.

❦ Whipped cream can be used as the base of an herbal infusion to treat dry skin. Let the chopped, dried herbs of your choice (try lavender, sage, rosemary, rose petals, or calendula) soak in heavy cream for at least 30 minutes. Then whip the cream and apply to the face. Leave on for 5 to 10 minutes. Rinse with a toning liquid (lemon juice, vinegar, or witch hazel mixed with an equal amount of water). Moisturize as usual.

❦ Buttermilk, heavy cream, yogurt, honey, mashed avocado or avocado oil, lanolin, and oils such as wheat germ, sesame, coconut, olive, canola, almond, apricot, and citrus are all natural moisturizers. Experiment with them (doing skin tests first to check for negative reactions; see page 97) in combination with various herbs; astringents such as lemon juice or witch hazel; and exfoliants such as oats, couscous, or mashed apple, pineapple, or strawberries.

Cucumber Facial

Use this facial to soothe and cleanse the skin. Some say cucumbers with lemon juice erase freckles. The recipe is certainly astringent. Cukes also contain a hormone thought to work against wrinkles. For best effect, apply after a shower or facial steaming. Be sure the skin is clean before you apply the mask. Do a skin test (see page 97) to check for any sensitivities you may have.

2-inch chunk fresh cucumber, seeded and pureed
1 teaspoon lemon juice
1 teaspoon witch hazel
1 egg white
2 tablespoons cream or plain yogurt
(optional; for dry skin)
2 teaspoons nonfat powdered milk
(optional; for normal skin)

Briefly puree all the ingredients in a blender. Apply to the face, avoiding the area around your eyes, and let sit until nearly dry, about 20 to 30 minutes. Rinse well with warm water.

Cucumber
(*Cucumis sativus*)

SHAMPOOS & REMEDIAL HAIR CARE

❦ A well-balanced diet is necessary for healthy hair. Poor nutrition, especially protein deficiencies, can lead to thinning, dull, dry hair (usually reversible with a return to good eating).

❦ The yucca plant contains saponins suitable for shampoo. Chop the roots and mix with warm water to make suds. Native Americans who had the yucca plant available to them used soapweed (*Yucca glauca*) to make a shampoo that was especially popular in certain marriage ceremonies where the couple might shampoo each other's hair.

❦ Soapwort is another natural shampoo. Chop the dried root and mix with warm water. While not highly sudsing, it works well to cleanse the hair.

❦ Some health food stores carry soapbark chips, from a Chilean evergreen, that can be mixed with warm water and used as a shampoo.

❦ Decoct quince seeds, about 1 ounce to 1 cup boiling water. Let sit for 1 hour, then strain. This mucilaginous decoction can be used for hair care. In the past, some cultures considered it a remedy for baldness, probably because of the fuzzy quince skin, denoting a sympathetic cure under the doctrine of signatures.

❦ Some Native American tribes believed that rubbing the head with yarrow oil would stop hair from thinning.

❦ A sassafras bark shampoo is said to kill head lice.

❦ Use arrowroot powder as a dry shampoo when you're in a hurry or traveling. Simply sprinkle the powder near your scalp and brush your hair clean.

❦ Add a strained herbal infusion (1 tablespoon dried herb per 1 cup boiling water, steeped for at least 30 minutes) to flaked or liquid Castile soap to make a quick version of an herbal shampoo. Because Castile soap is olive oil based, be sure to rinse with a solution that includes at least a couple of tablespoons of vinegar or lemon juice for better pH balance.

Egg Shampoo

1 ounce fresh rosemary
1 pint hot water
1 egg

Steep the rosemary in the water for 20 minutes. Cool. Beat in the egg. Massage into the hair and rinse.

CONDITIONERS, RINSES & GELS

❦ "Take equal parts of castor oil and alcohol, about a pint of each, and add citronella, bergamot, and lavender or other aromatics of your choice for scent. Color with alkanet root [henna] and apply as a hair oil." (UNPUBLISHED RECIPE BOOK, C. 1850)

❦ Rose Water: Take a peck of rose petals, freshly picked, and simmer in 1 quart water over a slow fire until the liquid is reduced by one-half. Strain and bottle, leaving uncapped for 3 days, then cap the bottle. Use as a hair rinse or to scent cosmetics or salves.

❦ Herbs used to treat dandruff include burdock root, chamomile, clary sage, comfrey, elder flowers, eucalyptus, horsetail, lavender, peppermint, rosemary, sage, southernwood, stinging nettles, tea tree oil, and thyme. After shampooing, the infused or decocted herb is rubbed into the scalp, then rinsed briefly.

❦ Jewelweed was discovered by Native Americans and adopted by early settlers as a remedy for dandruff, athlete's foot, poison ivy, and insect bites and stings (see Chapter 3). As a dandruff treatment, take the juice from the swollen nodes and rub it into the scalp, then rinse with water.

❦ To cure dandruff, after shampooing rinse the scalp and hair with a solution of one part apple cider vinegar and two parts water.

❦ Infused chamomile or catmint can be used to treat a young child's scalp for cradle cap. Rub the infusion into the scalp after shampooing, scrub briskly with

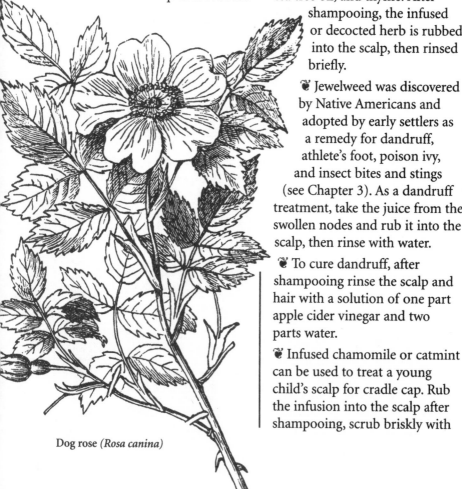

Dog rose (*Rosa canina*)

a washcloth or comb with a fine-toothed child's comb, and rinse.

❦ To stimulate the scalp and reduce hair loss, massage with an infusion of stinging nettles, ginger, thyme, parsley, or cloves in olive oil.

❦ Conditioning herbs for dry hair include burdock root, elder flowers, marshmallow, parsley, sage, and stinging nettles. Of these, many women prefer sage for its sweet fragrance.

❦ Conditioning herbs for oily hair include bee balm, calendula (marigold), lavender, any of the mints, rosemary, southernwood, and yarrow. For fragrance, many women prefer lavender, the mints, or rosemary.

❦ Add a tablespoon of apple cider vinegar to your rinse water to help remove shampoo residue or balance hard water conditions.

❦ Lemon juice, added to your rinse water, gives highlights to blond hair and helps reduce oiliness.

❦ To cover gray hair in brunets, concoct rinses made with black tea, rosemary, instant coffee, sage, or oregano, alone or in combination. Make a strained, infused tea of the chosen ingredients and pour over the hair, catching the rinse water in a basin and reapplying it repeatedly.

❦ To restore the natural color of brown hair, make a rinse of leeks. Boil a few leeks in water for 20

Brunet Booster

This solution helps cure dandruff, leaves hair shiny, and fades gray.

2 cups fresh sage
1 cup fresh rosemary
2 teaspoons apple cider
  vinegar

Place the sage and rosemary in a 6-quart pot and cover with water. Bring to a boil, then reduce the heat to barely a simmer. Simmer, covered, for up to 6 hours, making sure the water does not boil off. Remove from the heat and let steep overnight.

Strain the herbs out and add enough water to the strong tea that remains to make 5 cups. Add the vinegar and bottle.

Use this rinse after you wash your hair, rubbing it thoroughly into your scalp. Barely rinse it, so that some remains on your hair.

minutes, then strain out the solids. Use the water as a final hair rinse.

❦ The hulls of black walnuts can be decocted or pressed to make a dark hair color to cover gray. Like henna, this stains the skin, so use with caution. Do a skin test first (see page 97).

❦ For redheads, make a hair rinse of green tea to enhance your natural color and add shine.

❦ To make hair shinier, brunets should rinse with an infusion of rosemary, stinging nettles, sage, raspberry leaves, or elderberries. Blonds can use chamomile, yarrow, calendula, or mullein flowers. Redheads can go either way, depending on the lightness or darkness of their hair.

❦ According to the doctrine of signatures, Native Americans used the maidenhair fern in a hair rinse as an early equivalent of a conditioner.

❦ Use the gel of the aloe vera plant, straight from the leaf, as a setting gel or mousse for styling or curling your hair. Leave on, dry your hair, and brush.

❦ Use beer as a setting lotion. Even the professional salons do it.

❦ Egg is nourishing to hair, resupplying protein where it may be lacking in brittle or dried-out hair. Even better is mayonnaise, which contains egg for protein and vinegar for luster and bounce.

Use either as a conditioner, letting it remain on the hair for a few minutes, then rinsing well with warm water. You can also whip egg whites for use as a protein-based mousse for styling.

❦ Decoct quince seeds or flax seeds in water, let thicken, and use as a setting gel.

❦ For swimmers, especially blonds, who are exposed to chlorinated water on a regular basis, rinse the hair with tomato juice after swimming. This helps remove the chlorine and prevents that greenish tinge it can impart to light-colored hair.

❦ To Promote Hair Growth: "Equal quantities of olive-oil and spirit of rosemary; a few drops of oil of nutmeg. Mix the ingredients together, rub the roots of the hair every night with a little of this liniment, and the growth of it will very soon sensibly increase." (MB)

∞○∞

Comet, shake out your locks and let them flare
Across the startled heaven of my soul!
Pluck out the hairpins, Sue, and let her roll!
Don't be so stingy with your blooming hair.

— DONALD ROBERT PERRY MARQUIS (1878–1937)

∞○∞

Maidenhair fern
(*Adiantum* spp.)

A Good Night's Sleep

Not every fragrant herb is suitable to rest your head upon. Some aromas, such as that of rosemary, may be pleasing for some and headache breeders for others. If you give away a sleep pillow, dream pillow, or fragrant eye mask, be sure to identify what's in it.

Sleep pillows generally include insomnia-combating herbs such as hops, lavender, chamomile, Our Lady's bedstraw (*Galium verum*, reputed to have been used in the cradle or manger for baby Jesus), thyme, lemon verbena, lemon balm, and sweet marjoram. These can be used singly or combined. Abraham Lincoln used a pillow of hops to help prevent insomnia. If hops are used, they should be replaced every three to six months because their smell turns fetid with time and can cause headaches or — you guessed it — insomnia! Dream pillows are used to dispel nightmares and make sweet dreams more vivid.

Some herbalists warn against using any artemisia other than mugwort in sleep or dream pillows. Tansy, commercial potpourris, French marigolds, strong fragrance oils, and bay leaves also are cautioned against. With the exception of lavender, which can be used fresh because it won't mold, all ingredients should be well dried.

Pillows for Peaceful Nights

To make a sleep or dream pillow, make an inner cloth envelope of cheesecloth or tulle for the herbs.

Sleep Pillow
½ cup chamomile flowers
½ cup rosemary leaves
½ cup pine needles
1 cup lavender flowers
2 tablespoons lemon verbena
  leaves
1 tablespoon pinhead orrisroot
  (a stabilizer)
½ teaspoon oil of lavender

Dream Pillow
½ cup mugwort leaves
½ cup lavender flowers
½ cup spearmint or peppermint
  leaves
2 tablespoons thyme leaves
2 tablespoons rosemary leaves
1 tablespoon pinhead orrisroot
  (a stabilizer)

Combine ingredients and fill cloth envelope. Slip it inside any washable pillowcase.

INSOMNIA & DISTURBED SLEEP

First calm thyself. If gardening or another relaxing activity doesn't calm your nerves and make you sleep well, try a tea (really a tisane, from the Greek for "medicinal brew") of chamomile, basil, marjoram, or lavender. Most herbal sleeping aids are simple infusions made by pouring boiling water over leaves and flowers, then letting them steep for five minutes. Use about 1 ounce fresh herbs (half of that if dried) for every 2 to 3 cups water in a prewarmed crockery teapot. Some recipes call for 1 teaspoon dried herbs or 3 teaspoons fresh herbs per cup, plus 1 teaspoon for the pot. If you plan to add ice, double the quantity of herbs. Before adding seeds (anise or dill), crush them with a mortar and pestle.

❦ Do not eat your final meal late in the evening, and keep the meal light.

❦ Eating lettuce with your dinner is supposed to be calming, helping you to sleep and have pleasant dreams. Some say you should not have vinegar with your lettuce. Both lettuce and cucumbers are ruled by the moon, which some say make them good sleep remedies.

❦ Mandarin oranges are soporifics, so consider adding them to your evening meal.

❦ Strew lavender in the linen closet to scent your bed sheets with this mildly narcotic herb.

❦ Sprinkle infusions of dill on your pillowcases and quickly iron them dry or fluff them in a clothes dryer.

❦ Native American tea ingredients for insomnia included lady's slipper (decocted), yarrow, mullein, hops, and purslane (also decocted).

❦ Bee balm tea acts as a mild sedative, calming the nerves and aiding sleep. Take an infusion of 2 teaspoons chopped fresh leaves in 1 cup boiling water. Dried leaves will do, but fresh ones are more potent.

❦ A tea of elderberry flowers (*Sambucus nigra*) is considered sleep inducing and relaxing to the nerves. (**Caution!** Avoid if pregnant.)

❦ Catnip tea and chamomile tea are used for both nervous conditions and insomnia in infants and adults.

❦ For young babies having trouble sleeping, try a warm bath with a couple of drops of chamomile oil added. Lavender oil (one part lavender to two parts chamomile) can be included for a relaxing aroma. (See other aromatic baths earlier in this chapter.)

❦ Native Americans reportedly ate raw onions to induce sleep.

❦ Native Americans also made a sleep syrup from poppy seeds and flowers or a tea from poppy heads decocted in water.

❦ Native Americans used jimsonweed poultices for extreme insomnia. This and henbane extract were considered alternatives to opium.

❦ Dill will lull cranky babies to sleep. Add a dill infusion to the bath, sprinkle the infusion on a baby's blanket, or use it as a hair rinse.

❦ Sage is considered a "ghost medicine," used to prevent nightmares. Burn it as incense in the bedroom or strew it on the floor or in the bed.

❦ "To procure sleep, wash the head in a decoction of dill seed, and smell of it frequently." (LIA)

❦ Valerian (sometimes called tobacco plant or all-heal) tea or capsules are frequently mentioned as a primary aid for those having trouble sleeping. Some people find the smell of valerian tea unpleasant and the taste bitter, so they choose to take

Dill *(Anethum graveolens)*

valerian capsules instead. In infusions, 1 ounce of the roots in 1 pint boiling water is a common recipe, consumed by the wineglass as needed. (**Caution!** Too high a dose may lead to headaches, dizziness, depression, muscle spasms, or nausea.) Preliminary studies seem to indicate that valerian does not react adversely in combination with alcohol or produce undesirable "morning after" effects.

❦ Lady's slipper "promotes sleep, and allays the headache. Dose, one tea-spoonful in warm water, adding a little sugar." (LIA)

❦ Gotu kola (*Hydrocotyle asiatica*) is sold in health food stores and often used as a mild sedative for sleeping problems. The Food and Drug Administration (FDA) categorizes it as an herb of "undefined safety," meaning that little is known about it.

❦ "For Vigilia, or Inability to Sleep: Apply to the forehead, for two hours, cloths four times doubled, dipped in cold water. I have known this applied to a lying-in woman and her life saved thereby.... Drink no green tea in the afternoon." (JW)

❦ Europeans often drink passionflower tea for sleeplessness.

Chapter 8

Caution & Common Sense

Good health and good sense are two of life's greatest blessings.

— *PUBLILIUS SYRUS (C. 42 B.C.)*

atural" or "plant-based" doesn't necessarily mean harmless. With any herbal remedy, proceed with caution and moderation. Be sure you have correctly identified your plant materials. When in doubt, check with an expert, whether it is a trained botanist who knows how to gather plants from the wild, a gardener who has grown the plant you seek, or the health food store or pharmacy from which you buy the ingredient. Use the proper Latin name for the herb to avoid possible confusion with common names (see Appendix I). Consider growing your own, again being sure to specify the Latin name when obtaining seeds.

For safety, consult a qualified health practitioner before proceeding with any internal remedies, especially if you are pregnant, nursing, or have other insinuating conditions such as high blood pressure or diabetes. For children's doses, see pages 113–114. Some remedies are marked as particularly safe for children. Otherwise, use extra caution before treating a child with an adult remedy.

Comfrey (*Symphytum officinale*)

G E N E R A L   C A U T I O N S

In general, use home remedies for common, familiar, and short-term complaints such as a sore throat, cold, headache, cough, or stomachache. As with any condition, if symptoms persist or become worse, consult your doctor. Do not ingest large quantities of any home remedy. Even if the herb itself is quite safe, your source may contain contaminants that are unknown to you. (Learn as much as you can about where your ingredients come from.) Prolonged use of home remedies could put you at risk.

If you are under a doctor's care for any reason; if you are nursing, pregnant, or trying to conceive; if you have a family history or personal history of any medical condition such as diabetes, heart trouble, high blood pressure, or other insinuating factors; or if you are taking any medications, let your doctor know what you're considering in the way of self-treatment, even if it's only a cup of medicinal tea. Some orthodox medicines interact (sometimes unfavorably) with certain herbs. Your doctor may have important advice for you pertaining to your particular medical history or condition and the use of that remedy.

Do not discontinue traditional prescribed medicines or substitute home remedies for them without consulting your doctor.

Just because a tea or remedy is sold under a name that implies it's good for certain symptoms, that doesn't mean it's safe or there's any scientific proof to back that implication. Always use your own knowledge and judgment. Find out as much as you can about any remedy you plan to use, especially if you are contemplating long-term use.

Never ingest essential oils, except possibly under professional advice.

Be sure to check on children's doses (see the chart on page 114).

The very elderly or very sick may need a decreased dose. Physical debilitation as a result of long-term illness should be considered as well.

For remedies intended for external use, you may want to perform a patch test on your inner arm to check for adverse reactions (see page 97). If your skin reacts adversely, do not use them even aromatically. A skin test can sometimes warn of negative reactions to herbs intended for internal use as well.

Be aware of remedies with sedative actions and use them with respect. Do not drive or operate machinery after taking sedative herbs. In some cases, excesses of sedative herbs can lead to depressed respiratory or cardiac function, depression of the thyroid, or melancholy. Large doses sometimes lead to insomnia.

MAKING YOUR OWN REMEDIES

❦ Don't dilute tinctures or essential oils as a substitute for infusions or decoctions. You're apt to get too high a dose.

❦ Loose herbs or teas, sold without the packaging of a particular manufacturer, are more likely to contain contaminants than prepackaged versions. Although the loose form may be cheaper, it's often of poorer quality. Even among the prepackaged versions, there's a wide range of quality. Read the ingredients on the package and find out as much as you can about the source.

❦ With essential oils and tinctures, the more expensive versions are often purer. Again, know your sources and seek to identify (using the Latin names where applicable) exactly what's in a particular remedy.

❦ When making infusions, decoctions, or other heated remedies, don't use metal pans or containers, such as aluminum or cast-iron cookware. Instead, choose a heat-resistant glass such as Pyrex. Enamel-coated pans are safe to use as long as the enamel is not pitted, chipped, or worn away. For most infusions that require only brief simmering, stainless steel is safe. Similarly, nylon sieves are better than metal ones for straining the plant parts from the liquid.

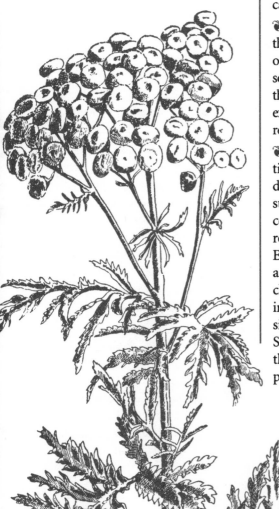

Tansy
(*Tanacetum vulgare*)

IF YOU ARE PREGNANT

❦ Herbs such as cinnamon, sage, nutmeg, and fennel, common in everyday cooking, are safe in normal doses. In therapeutic doses, however, they could pose problems for pregnant women because they are uterine stimulants. Let common sense be your guide, keep your health practitioner informed of any remedies you are considering, and seek expert advice when in doubt.

❦ Find out whether herbs are uterine stimulants or relaxants and respect that knowledge. A qualified practitioner might recommend a tea containing a uterine stimulant once labor has begun, but it could be unwise to consume that same tea during your first trimester of pregnancy or, in some cases, even later in pregnancy. Report any spotting or bleeding to your health practitioner immediately.

❦ Pregnant women should not take herbs containing salicin (an aspirinlike compound found, for example, in many poplar and willow barks) because of the risks associated with aspirin and birth defects or Reye's syndrome.

❦ When considering home remedies for ills common to pregnancy, such as morning sickness or constipation, or other common ailments such as colds and flu, be sure to assess the actions of the ingredients and how they may affect you and the fetus. For example, although goldenseal is often recommended for colds, it is not recommended during pregnancy because it is also a uterine stimulant.

CHILDREN'S DOSES

Not all herbal remedies are suitable for children. Even those that are commonly recommended for children (such as agrimony, burdock, chamomile, catnip, dill, elder flower, eyebright, fennel, licorice, linden, plantain, and white horehound, to name a few) should be used in children's doses, based on the age and/or weight of the child.

❦ As with any remedy, start slowly and with small quantities, carefully noting any reactions.

❦ If you are nursing, keep in mind that any remedy you ingest is being passed on to the infant through your breast milk.

❦ Where tinctures are called for, use ones with a nonalcoholic base, especially for infants.

❦ Do not hesitate to consult a doctor, and never use any remedy on a long-term basis without a doctor's knowledge.

❦ Children under 16 should not take herbs containing salicin (an aspirinlike compound found, for example, in many poplar and willow barks) because of the risks associated with aspirin and birth defects or Reye's syndrome.

❦ For constipation, never use strong laxatives or purgatives for children. Fennel, dill, and chamomile are often suggested instead.

❦ Keep all remedies out of children's reach. If a remedy must be refrigerated, use a childproof container.

❦ For fever, catmint, elder flower, or yarrow teas are recommended.

❦ For children's earaches, various remedies such as olive oil with goldenseal, wormwood, or other herbs are sometimes suggested as eardrops.

Children's Dosage Guide

Age (years)	Approximate Weight (pounds)	Dose (fraction of adult dose)*
0 to ½	3 to 18	about $\frac{1}{20}$
½ to 1	10 to 25	$\frac{1}{20}$ to $\frac{1}{5}$
1 to 3	20 to 35	$\frac{1}{10}$ to $\frac{1}{5}$
3 to 5	30 to 50	$\frac{1}{5}$ to $\frac{1}{4}$
5 to 7	35 to 60	$\frac{3}{10}$ to $\frac{1}{3}$
7 to 9	45 to 70	$\frac{2}{5}$ to $\frac{1}{2}$
9 to 11	55 to 85	$\frac{1}{5}$ to $\frac{3}{5}$
11 to 13	65 to 95	$\frac{3}{5}$ to full dose
13 to 15	85 to 110	$\frac{4}{5}$ to full dose
15 and up	95 and up	Full dose

* For a child whose weight is still very slight by comparison with the approximate weights given for that age, give a lesser dose based on a younger child of similar weight. Similarly, children who are above the average weight for their age can usually tolerate the dose for an older child of that weight. No distinction is made here between girls' and boys' weights; the chart applies to both sexes. (This chart is not intended as a standard for healthy weight gain at various ages.)

An Alphabetical Guide to Medicinal Herbs & Other Ingredients

*D*o not assume from any of the recommendations in this book that if no cautions are listed for a particular ingredient, it is safe. In the United States, the Food and Drug Administration's highest rating for any herb is that it is "generally recognized as safe," which may suggest only that possible dangers are as yet unknown. Similarly, the lack of cautions listed here may indicate a lack of information available on that herb. Furthermore, even herbs considered generally safe for most people may cause allergic or other reactions in some people. As with any remedy, your own careful research, observations, and consultation with experts are your best guide.

Agrimony (*Agrimonia* spp., most notably *A. eupatoria* or, in China, *A. pilosa;* also called cocklebur, church steeples, or stickwort). The aerial parts are astringent, tannic, bitter, and diuretic. Sometimes used to stop bleeding or for children's intestinal distress. (**Caution!** Do not use if constipated.)

Alfalfa (*Medicago sativa;* also called Spanish clover, purple medick, or lucerne). A perennial legume. The aerial parts can be used for nourishment and as a digestive tonic. Contains carotene. Sometimes suggested as a daily tea (in moderation) for anemia or for toning the system during pregnancy or menopause.

Alliums (*Allium* spp., especially *A. sativum*). Garlic, onions, scallions, shallots, and, to a lesser degree, chives, which are rich in sulfur compounds and have antibacterial qualities. Historically, the concentric layers of the onion were believed to draw contagious diseases from the patient into the bulb. Thus, an onion was often hung in a sickroom. Native Americans used wild onions and wild leeks for coughs and colds. Today many mouthwashes and throat lozenges include a synthetic equivalent of the active bacteria-killing property in onion juice. See also Garlic.

Allspice (*Pimenta officinalis*). The dried berries are ground as a spice. Do not ingest allspice oil (which contains a substance called eugenol); it is highly concentrated and can cause nausea. The oil is sometimes used topically as a pain reliever, such as for toothache, but do not swallow it. The powder can be used for externally applied infusions or poultices. Allspice is an antioxidant with certain anticancer actions, but eugenol has been linked with promoting cancer growth.

Aloe vera (*Aloe vera*). A member of the Liliaceae family. A gel from the leaves of the plant may be used externally for inflammations or mild burns and sunburns. Best not to use internally, as its laxative chemicals are very strong. It's also a uterine stimulant.

Angelica (*Angelica archangelica*). The leaves or roots are used as a diuretic, expectorant, antispasmodic, and carminative. Benedictine (the liqueur) contains angelica. The stalks are sometimes candied. As a warming digestive tonic, it's sometimes used for children's respiratory ills. (**Cautions!** Contains psoralens, which cause a rash in some people upon exposure to the sun. The Chinese form, *A. sinensis* [dang gui], has possible links with miscarriage. Both forms are uterine stimulants; don't use if pregnant. Avoid if diabetic. Don't harvest your own, as it's easily confused with water hemlock [*Cicuta maculata* and others]. Do not confuse with wild angelica [*A. atropurpurea*].)

Anise (*Pimpinella anisum*). An expectorant and antiseptic. The essential oil (not to be ingested) and the seeds are the most commonly used parts.

Arnica (*Arnica montana;* also called leopard's bane or wolfsbane). An aromatic made from the flowers and a traditional homeopathic remedy available commercially in tablets, creams, or ointments. Often used for calming after a minor accident or shock. Arnica cream also is used for sprains or bruises and sometimes for rheumatism. (**Cautions!** In homeopathic doses, the amount ingested is very small, but taken internally in significant amounts, arnica is toxic. It contains vasoactive constituents [affecting the blood vessels]. Do not use on broken skin; it can be an irritant. Some herbals recommend avoiding arnica altogether, especially without expert medical advice.)

Balm of Gilead (*Populus gileadensis* or *P. balsamifera*). The buds are used as an antiseptic and expectorant. Often used for throat troubles and bronchial infections. Contains salicin. (**Caution!** Not for use by pregnant women or children under 16 because of the risks associated with aspirin [salicin] and birth defects or Reye's syndrome.)

Barberry (*Berberis vulgaris*). The bark is decocted and used to stimulate the flow of bile and to ease congestion of the liver. A bitter laxative. (**Cautions!** Do not use in pregnancy. Do not confuse with bearberry or bayberry.)

Basil (*Ocimum basilicum*). The aerial parts are used as an antiseptic and anti-depressant. (**Caution!** Avoid the essential oil, even externally, if pregnant.)

Bayberry (*Myrica cerifera*; also called waxberry, wax myrtle, or candleberry). The dried root is used as an astringent, circulatory stimulant, throat remedy, diarrhea remedy, and topical wound treatment. A tannin, with myrinic acid in its resin. (**Caution!** Do not confuse with barberry or bearberry.)

Bearberry (*Arctostaphylos uva ursi*; also called mountain cranberry, uva ursi, or sandberry). The berries are astringent and antiseptic. Often used for urinary tract infections. (**Cautions!** Can produce nausea if taken in high doses. Avoid if kidneys are damaged. Do not confuse with barberry or bayberry.)

Bee balm. See Lemon balm. (**Caution!** Do not confuse with *Monarda didyma,* also called bee balm but not to be used medicinally.)

Benzoin (*Styrax benzoin*). The essential oil and gum are used as an expectorant and astringent. Available in tincture form and often used to season or stabilize liniments and other remedies.

Birthwort (*Aristolochia* spp.). Birthwort takes its genus name from the Greek words meaning "best for childbirth." Some assign it to the doctrine of signatures, saying the curved flower and base resemble a human fetus in the right position for birth. The Greeks, Romans, Arabs, Hindus, and American Indians used birthwort to aid parturition. U.S. varieties are found in the warmer regions only and include Virginia snakeroot (the root being good for snakebite, some say) and pelican flower.

Blackberry (*Rubus occidentalis*). The leaves and root bark are variously used in infusions or decoctions, especially to treat diarrhea.

Black cohosh (*Cimicifuga racemosa*; also called squawroot, rattleweed, rattletop, bugbane, or black snakeroot). The root is used as an antispasmodic and uterine stimulant; sometimes suggested to bring on the menses.

Contains estrogenic substances. (**Caution!** Avoid in pregnancy. Contains saponins, which should not be used on broken skin, as they can dissolve red blood cells.)

Black haw (*Viburnum prunifolium*). The bark contains salicin and is decocted and used to ease menstrual cramps. A uterine relaxant, sedative, and anti-inflammatory. (**Caution!** Not for use by pregnant women or children under 16 because of the risks associated with aspirin [salicin] and birth defects or Reye's syndrome.)

Blessed thistle (*Cnicus benedictus;* also called holy thistle). A purgative, promotes sweating, and sometimes used for jaundice and vertigo. An astringent and digestive stimulant.

Blue cohosh (*Caulophyllum thalictroides;* also called squawroot, papooseroot, or blue ginseng). The rhizomes and roots are used, especially for dysmenorrhea. An antispasmodic tonic for the reproductive system. (**Cautions!** Should not be used in pregnancy, at least until labor has commenced, and then only under professional advice. Can lower blood pressure; seek medical advice pertaining to this attribute. Contains saponins, which should not be used on broken skin, as they can dissolve red blood cells.)

Boneset. See Comfrey, Feverwort, and Gravelroot.

Borage (*Borago officinalis*). The leaves and flowers are an expectorant, antirheumatic, adrenal stimulant, and diuretic. They also promote lactation. The seeds were once suggested for skin inflammations, joint aches, and to regulate the bowels. (**Cautions!** Restricted in some countries. Avoid long-term use. Some recent studies suggest that borage should be avoided altogether, especially for internal use, because of a possible connection with liver damage [see Comfrey].)

Burdock (*Arctium lappa;* also called beggar's-buttons or thorny burr). A common roadside plant in North America. The dried root is the most commonly used part, but the leaves are often used as well. Fresh parts contain antibiotic substances. Both the root and the aerial parts are a diuretic, a mild laxative, and generally cleansing to the system. Burdock is most commonly suggested for releasing toxins from the body. Also used externally for boils, sores, eczema, and other skin inflammations. (**Caution!** Excessive doses are to be avoided. Many herbalists recommend starting slowly, then working up as appropriate.)

Burnet. See Greater burnet.

Butternut (*Juglans cinerea;* also called white walnut). The bark of the tree is decocted as a stimulating laxative; sometimes suggested for children. Stimulates the flow of bile from the liver.

Cabbage (*Brassica oleracea*). The leaves of the common cabbage can be used as a poultice, as they are anti-inflammatory, antibacterial, and antirheumatic. Internally, they are a liver decongestant. (**Caution!** Tends to depress thyroid function [as do all members of the cabbage and mustard family]. Avoid where thyroid levels are low.)

Calendula (*Calendula officinalis*; also called pot marigold, marybud, or marigold). In the purest form, just the petals are used. Commercial dried forms generally include the flower heads. The leaves are sometimes used for poultices. An astringent, antiseptic, and anti-inflammatory. The essential oil is antifungal. (**Cautions!** Do not confuse this with the French marigold [*Tagetes patula*], used for insecticides, herbicides, and wart removal. As with any essential oil, do not ingest.)

Camphor (*Cinnamomum camphora*; sometimes spelled camphire). A volatile crystalline compound from camphor tree wood (or synthesized). Used as an insect repellent, both a stimulant and a sedative, an expectorant, and a diaphoretic (producing perspiration). (**Caution!** Some herbals suggest avoiding this altogether, especially internally.)

Caraway (*Carum carvi*). A fatty oil and tannin, a stimulating expectorant, and an antispasmodic. The seeds are used as a digestive stimulant and antiseptic and sometimes sugared as "comfits."

Castor oil (*Racinis communis*). The oil comes from the seeds of the castor-oil plant and is used for bowel regularity and as a cure-all and spring tonic.

Catmint, catnip (*Nepeta cataria*). The aerial parts are used as a digestive stimulant, to produce perspiration, to reduce fever, to reduce upper respiratory congestion, and as an antispasmodic and astringent. Often suggested for children with colds, earaches, sinus trouble, or congestion.

Cayenne pepper (*Capsicum minimum* or *C. frutescens*; also called chili, red pepper, or bird pepper). Available both in pods and powdered, the dried fruits of cayenne are a powerful circulatory stimulant and often suggested for warming or counterirritant uses (externally in poultices or salves) in cases of joint inflammation. Cayenne compresses should be monitored carefully to make sure skin does not blister or become irritated. Some commercial creams containing capsaicin, the alkaloid constituent of cayenne, are used for arthritis, shingles, diabetic foot pains, and other external uses. Cayenne also produces perspiration, stimulates gastric secretions, and is antiseptic. (**Cautions!** Cayenne can be severely irritating to the eyes, open wounds, and mucous membranes. Avoid if you have a history of ulcers or other stomach problems or if you are pregnant or nursing. Avoid using the seeds, which can be toxic.)

Celandine (*Chelidonium majus*; also called greater celandine, garden celandine, or swallowwort). Pliny the Elder said it bloomed when the swallows arrived and its petals dropped when they left; the yellow juice was considered good for jaundice, the throat, and failing eyesight. The Medicines Act of 1968 restricted the sale of this herb to medical herbalists trained in its use. The leaves are anti-inflammatory, diuretic, laxative, and antispasmodic; generally used for cleansing the liver and bowels. (**Cautions!** Best left to the professionals, even for external use. Poisonous in large doses. Avoid in pregnancy.)

Celery (*Apium graveolens;* also called smallage). The seed is used to stimulate milk flow and as a urinary antiseptic and diuretic, uterine stimulant, and digestive tonic. (**Cautions!** Avoid if pregnant. The essential oil is distilled from the seed and is highly potent; avoid it, even externally, during pregnancy, as it's a uterine stimulant. The seed sold horticulturally is often treated with fungicides and should not be used medicinally.)

Chamomile, German (*Matricaria recutita;* also called wild chamomile or ground apple). The Latin name *Matricaria* hints of its gynecological uses as a uterine stimulant. The homeopathic Chamomilla remedy is given for menstrual pain and during labor, as well as for teething or colicky babies. Because of its mildness, chamomile is one of the most widely suggested remedies for children and has the U.S. Food and Drug Administration's highest plant categorization: "generally recognized as safe." The dried flowers are an anti-inflammatory, antispasmodic, and mild sedative (without being depressing). They are useful for fever management and as an inhalant for congestion and are calming to the digestive tract and nerves. (**Cautions!** The essential oil is a uterine stimulant; avoid if pregnant. Some people experience dermatitis from contact with chamomile. Also, those prone to ragweed or other daisy family allergies may experience allergic reactions to chamomile, though rarely to German chamomile.)

Chamomile, Roman (*Anthemis nobilis* or *Chamaemelum nobile*). The "true," or perennial, chamomile. This is herbalists' and gardeners' favored version, although it and German chamomile are virtually identical for medicinal use. See Chamomile, German, for actions and cautions.

Chaste berry (*Vitex agnus-castus*). A hormone stimulant. (**Caution!** Large quantities have been known to cause itching.)

Chickweed (*Stellaria media*). The aerial parts are antirheumatic, astringent, and demulcent. Often suggested to heal wounds and soothe itchy skin.

Cilantro (*Coriandrum sativum;* also called Chinese parsley). The seeds of cilantro are known as coriander; the leaves are called cilantro. Both are used as medicinals. Antioxidant, antibacterial, and anti-inflammatory. Used as a digestive aid for flatulence and diarrhea. A weak tea of the leaves can be given to babies for colic; stronger teas are used in adults for arthritis. The seeds are sometimes used in salves and ointments for healing wounds or easing joint pain.

Cinnamon (*Cinnamomum zeylanicum*). The dried inner bark of a tree. A warming digestive, antispasmodic, and antiseptic. Both the bark and the essential oil are uterine stimulants, so, for example, cinnamon oil would *not* be a good massage oil for a woman in early pregnancy, but it might be just the thing (well diluted in some other oil) for menstrual cramps. (**Cautions!** Avoid therapeutic doses in pregnancy because of possible uterine stimulation.

Never ingest the essential oil, which could cause kidney damage and vomiting. Can be irritating to the skin.)

Clary (*Salvia sclarea;* also called clary sage). The aerial parts are used as a uterine stimulant, nerve tonic, and digestive aid. (**Cautions!** Not for use in pregnancy. Toxic in high doses and may cause headaches.) See also Sage.

Clove (*Syzygium aromaticum*). The essential oil and flower buds are used for aromatic and pain-suppressing functions. An antiseptic, antispasmodic, and stimulant. Can alleviate vomiting. (**Cautions!** Don't ingest clove oil. Discontinue its use on the skin if a rash develops. Don't smoke cloves in any form, as they release carcinogens.)

Colicroot. See Wild yam.

Comfrey (*Symphytum officinale;* also called backwort, bruisewort, boneset, or knitback). The leaves and roots are used externally in poultices for bruises and broken bones. In the 1970s, comfrey became very popular for coughs, digestive disorders, and cancer. However, it was later discovered that the pyrrolizidine alkaloids (PAs) in comfrey, especially in the roots and new leaves, are linked with liver toxicity and tumors. Until a PA-free version is developed, it may be best to steer clear of this old remedy. Comfrey's healing allantoins also are present in borage (*Borago officinalis*) and plantain (*Plantago major*). (**Cautions!** Do not use on dirty wounds because the healing action is so quick. Avoid for internal use. If you do use comfrey, the mature leaves, harvested late in the season, are less apt to contain the harmful PAs, and short-term use will minimize your exposure.)

Coneflower, purple. See Echinacea.

Coriander. See Cilantro.

Corn silk (*Zea mays*). The stigmas and styles are diuretic and soothing to the urinary tract.

Cowslip (*Primula veris, P. vulgaris,* or *P. officinalis*). Cowslips are almost indistinguishable from primroses, and both are used interchangeably as medicinals. The dried flowers are an expectorant, antispasmodic, and sedative. The roots contain salicin, an aspirinlike compound. (**Cautions!** Pregnant women and children under 16 should not take herbs containing salicin because of the risks associated with aspirin and birth defects or Reye's syndrome. Similarly, anyone using blood-thinning drugs should avoid this medicinal. Contains saponins, which should not be used on broken skin, as they can dissolve red blood cells.)

Cramp bark (*Viburnum opulus;* also called guelder rose or European cranberry). Cramp bark contains valeric acid, salicosides, tannin, and a resin. It is used locally as a muscle relaxant.

Curly dock. See Yellow dock.

Damask rose. See Rose.

Damiana (*Turnera diffusa aphrodisiaca*). The aerial parts are used. The variant Latin name suggests one of its reputed uses: stimulation of the reproductive system (especially male). Damiana also is a mild laxative, a urinary antiseptic, and restorative to the nerves.

Damson (*Damascenum* spp.). A purplish black oval plum. John Wesley prescribed preserved damsons to cure hiccups. Also used for respiratory ills and coughs.

Dandelion (*Taraxacum officinale;* also called lion's-tooth or fairy clock). The leaves are a digestive and gentle diuretic commonly used in spring tonics for cleansing the liver. The roots also are a diuretic and are used for cleansing the liver, gallstones, and joint and skin inflammations. The sap of the root is used locally for warts. (**Caution!** Children are sometimes taught that they can suck the "milk" of dandelions, which in moderation is relatively harmless but in large doses can cause diarrhea or vomiting. Beware of lawn chemicals as well.)

Dill (*Anethum graveolens*). The seeds are used, mashed and then infused, for stomach ills, colic, diarrhea, and flatulence. Antibacterial and carminative. (**Caution!** In rare cases, some people experience a skin rash from ingesting dill.)

Dock. See Yellow dock.

Echinacea (*Echinacea purpurea* or *E. angustifolia;* also called purple coneflower). The root is the most commonly used part of echinacea, although the flower can be used as well. It is fast becoming the number one herbal enhancer of the immune system, especially for colds, mucous infections, and kidney infections, although toxic effects have been reported. (**Cautions!** High doses may cause dizziness or nausea. Purity can be a problem in sources of echinacea; this is an easy one to consider growing yourself. Short-term use is advised.)

Elder (*Sambucus nigra;* also called black elder). The dried flowers are used for fever, as an expectorant, and as a diuretic. Very drying. The bark is a diuretic, purgative, and, in large doses, emetic. (**Caution!** Avoid the bark in pregnancy.)

Elecampane (*Inula helenium* or, in China, *I. japonica*). The roots and flowers are antibacterial, antifungal, and antiparasitic. They are used as an expectorant and a digestive stimulant.

Eucalyptus (*Eucalyptus globulus*). The leaves are highly antiseptic and are used for inflammations, as an expectorant, and in poultices. Eucalyptus also reduces blood sugar levels, is an antispasmodic, and has a reputation for expelling worms. (**Cautions!** Best used externally. Never ingest the oil, which is highly toxic even in small quantities. Avoid if you are insulin dependent, except with professional advice.)

Eyebright (*Euphrasia officinalis*). The aerial parts are used as an antiseptic, anti-phlegmatic, anti-inflammatory, eyewash, and gargle.

False unicorn root (*Chamaelirium luteum;* also called helonias root). The rhizome is used as a diuretic and uterine tonic and to cause vomiting. Stimulates ovarian hormones. (**Caution!** Contains saponins, which should not be used on broken skin, as they can dissolve red blood cells.)

Fennel (*Foeniculum vulgare*). The seeds and, less commonly, the roots are used, the latter mainly for urinary troubles. The essential oil is distilled from the seeds. Both are used as a diuretic, expectorant, and anti-inflammatory and to promote lactation and the menses. Often suggested for children or for nursing mothers with colicky babies. (**Cautions!** Avoid therapeutic doses if pregnant. Possible estrogenic effects. Don't harvest wild fennel; it closely resembles poison hemlock. Some herbals say to avoid the essential oil for children under six years old.)

Fenugreek (*Trigonella foenum-grecum*). The seeds are used as a nutritive, digestive, demulcent, and anti-inflammatory. They promote lactation, reduce blood sugar levels, stimulate the uterus, and may act as an aphrodisiac. The aerial parts are sometimes used as an antispasmodic. (**Cautions!** Avoid if you are insulin dependent, except with professional advice. Avoid if pregnant.)

Feverfew (*Tanacetum parthenium* or *Chrysanthemum parthenium;* also called featherfew or midsummer daisy). Some studies suggest that feverfew capsules can reduce the number and severity of migraine headaches. Only good-quality sources of feverfew leaves or tea contain its active ingredient, parthenolide, however. A uterine stimulant, digestive, and relaxant. (**Cautions!** Avoid if pregnant. Can cause mouth sores or lip ulcers. Avoid if taking blood thinners.)

Feverwort (*Eupatorium perfoliatum;* also called boneset, thoroughwort, hemp agrimony, or Indian sage). The aerial parts are a gentle laxative and expectorant. Being researched as an anticancer agent. Sometimes used for rheumatism, influenza, and to enhance the immune system. (**Cautions!** Not for young children. Do not eat fresh. High doses can cause nausea and vomiting.)

Flax, flaxseed. See Linseed.

Garlic (*Allium sativum*). Available in deodorized perles, or capsules, but fresh garlic is generally more effective unless you can't tolerate it for gastric or other reasons. Reduces cholesterol; selectively antipathogenic. Used as an antiseptic, vasodilator, expectorant, and antihistamine. Being studied for its potential in fighting heart disease, cancer, and AIDS. The U.S. Food and Drug Administration says garlic is "generally recognized as safe." (**Cautions!** Because of its anticlotting effects, anyone with hemophilia or other blood-clotting disorders should avoid garlic. Because of its reduction of blood sugar levels, diabetics should use it only with medical advice. Some people object to the garlic odor; others may have allergic reactions or skin inflammation from contact with or consumption of garlic. Some people experience gastric troubles from eating garlic. Some nursing mothers say it gives babies colic.)

Ginger (*Zingiber officinalis*). The so-called gingerroot is really a rhizome. It is a strong circulatory stimulant and vasodilator; used frequently for motion sickness, morning sickness, nausea, as an expectorant, and to relieve gas or colic. The essential oil can be used for rheumatic ills. The U.S. Food and Drug Administration says it's "generally recognized as safe." (**Cautions!** Some people develop heartburn from ginger. Doses of up to one gram have been used for morning sickness without apparent ill effects, but higher doses are discouraged in early pregnancy. Consult your doctor.)

Ginkgo (*Ginkgo biloba*; also called maidenhair tree). The seeds are antifungal, astringent, and antibacterial. The leaves are used as a circulatory stimulant that relaxes blood vessels; reputed to improve blood flow to the brain and improve memory and mental function. Ginkgo is being studied for use in Alzheimer's disease. (**Caution!** High doses of the seeds may cause headaches or skin problems.)

Ginseng (*Panax quinquefolium*, also called American ginseng or five-fingers; in China, *P. ginseng* or *P. notoginseng*; also, less commonly, *Eleutherococcus senticosus*, Siberian ginseng). The roots of these various ginsengs are used. The American versions are usually used for exhaustion or fever; the Chinese versions are more commonly suggested for reproductive energy or coronary ailments. (**Cautions!** Avoid taking any of the ginsengs with other stimulants such as cola, coffee, or caffeinated tea. Pregnant or nursing women should avoid *P. notoginseng* and also long-term or high doses of *P. ginseng*. Anyone with a history of hypertension or hyperactivity should avoid all the ginsengs, especially the Siberian version, which is even more stimulating than the others. Some herbals recommend no more than a three-week trial for children or active adults, reserving long-term use for the elderly who are beginning to experience debilitative or degenerative conditions such as Alzheimer's disease. Ginseng products are frequently adulterated with other substances, and some have been proven to contain no ginseng at all. Seek a reputable source and expect to pay a relatively high price for the real thing. Contains saponins, which should not be used on broken skin, as they can dissolve red blood cells.)

Goat's rue (*Galega officinalis*). The aerial parts are antispasmodic. (**Caution!** Avoid if diabetic; use only with a doctor's advice and monitoring of blood glucose.)

Goldenrod (*Solidago virgaurea*). Would you believe the aerial parts are a phlegm-reducing decongestant? So we're told. Also a sedative, astringent, and anti-inflammatory. Antiseptic to the urinary system, reducing blood pressure. (**Caution!** Avoid if you have trouble with low blood pressure.)

Goldenseal (*Hydrastis canadensis;* also called yellowroot or orangeroot). A traditional Native American medicinal, especially among the Cherokee and Iroquois. The rhizomes and roots are used for their astringent, digestive, and laxative actions; for the mucous membranes associated with respiratory trouble; and for heavy menses, premenstrual syndrome (PMS), or menopause. A uterine stimulant. (**Cautions!** Avoid if you are pregnant or have high blood pressure. Bloodroot is sometimes sold under the guise of goldenseal and has powerful laxative actions and serious side effects [nausea, dizziness, vomiting] at high doses. Seek a reputable source for goldenseal and avoid high doses, which have led to cardiac arrest and respiratory paralysis in animal studies. Typical recommended adult dose is only about ¼ teaspoon goldenseal diluted in 1 cup hot water. Long-term use could undermine the body's absorption of the B vitamins.)

Gotu kola (*Centella asiatica,* also called Indian pennywort; also the weaker *Hydrocotle asiatica,* which is more commonly available). The aerial parts are an adaptogenic tonic, relaxant, digestive, diuretic, and nervine. Short-term use is recommended. Use of the stronger *C. asiatica,* usually sold as capsules or extract, should be monitored by a professional. (**Cautions!** Sedative effects and possible skin rash have been associated with even the weaker version. High doses can cause itchy skin or headaches.)

Gravelroot (*Eupatorium purpureum,* also called joe-pye weed, queen of the meadow, or kidneyroot; *E. perfoliatum,* also called boneset or purple boneset; less commonly, *E. cannabium,* also called hemp agrimony, boneset, or feverwort). The rhizomes and roots are diuretic and soothing to the urinary system; sometimes suggested for urinary stones (as its name suggests), colds, menstrual ills (and to bring on the menses), or rheumatic disorders. A laxative, expectorant, and immune stimulant.

Greater burnet (*Sanguisorba officinalis;* also called burnet or garden burnet). The aerial parts are an astringent and tannin and are sometimes used for intestinal disorders.

Great mullein (*Verbascum thapsus;* also called lungwort, cow's lungwort, Aaron's rod, or lady's foxglove). Some recommend the flowers or leaves of great mullein for toothache, hemorrhoids, and diarrhea. Infusions of the leaves have been used for coughs, sore throats, chills, and fever. Promotes perspiration. An expectorant, mild diuretic, and astringent. Some use the infused oil for earaches. The U.S. Food and Drug Administration says it's "generally recognized as safe." (**Cautions!** The seeds are toxic. Tannins in mullein contain both carcinogens and anticancer agents; do not ingest if you have a history of cancer. Best used externally or as a gargle. Contains saponins, which should not be used on broken skin, as they can dissolve red blood cells.)

Ground ivy (*Nepeta hederacea* or *Glechoma hederacea;* also called alehoof or creeping Jenny). Leaves are astringent and anticatarrhal. Sometimes suggested for respiratory ills, to aid decongestion, for earaches, and as a gargle.

Heartsease (*Viola tricolor;* also called pansy, heartsease pansy, or herb trinity). The aerial parts are an expectorant, laxative, diuretic, and anti-inflammatory. Sometimes suggested for eczema or other skin problems or for bronchial ills. (**Caution!** Because of the saponin content, avoid very high doses, which could cause vomiting or nausea.) See also Sweet violet.

Henbane (*Hyoscyamus niger;* also called hog bean). The aerial parts are a sedative and antispasmodic. (**Caution!** Restricted to use by professional medical herbalists in the Medicines Act of 1968. Avoid except under expert advice.)

Honeysuckle (*Lonicera periclymenum* or *L. japonica*). The flowers and flower buds are a laxative, expectorant, and antispasmodic. (**Caution!** Honeysuckle berries are toxic and cause vomiting.)

Hops (*Humulus lupulus*). The flowers of the female plants, or strobiles, are used, either fresh or dried, for their antiseptic, sedative, digestive, and antispasmodic effects. (**Cautions!** Because hops are a mild depressant, they should be avoided by anyone plagued by depression. Fresh hops are suggested for insomnia, but the dried version can be stimulating. Some people experience skin rashes from direct contact with the fresh plant or its pollen. Harvesters often wear gloves. Japanese hops [*H. japonicus*] is an ornamental and is not to be used medicinally. Also, don't confuse common hops with wild hops [*Bryonia* spp.], which are poisonous if taken internally.)

Horehound, black (*Ballota nigra*). The aerial parts are a stimulant, antispasmodic, and antiemetic. Sometimes suggested for morning sickness.

Horehound, white (*Marrabium vulgare;* also spelled hoarhound). This is the horehound commonly used for coughs and congestion. The aerial parts are an expectorant, circulatory stimulant, relaxant, antispasmodic, and digestive. (**Cautions!** In large doses, horehound acts as a purgative and may precipitate an irregular heartbeat.)

Horse chestnut (*Aesculus hippocastanum*). The dried fruits (nuts) are astringent, diuretic, and anti-inflammatory. Used externally for hemorrhoids and varicose veins. Sometimes used internally for diarrhea and fever.

Horseradish (*Armoracia rusticana*). The root is used as a diuretic, powerful circulatory stimulant, and antiseptic. Stimulates stomach secretions. (**Cautions!** Tends to depress thyroid function [as do any of the cabbage and mustard family]. Avoid where thyroid levels are low. Can irritate the stomach.)

Horsetail (*Equisetum arvense;* also called shave grass or pewterwort). The aerial parts are an astringent, anti-inflammatory, and diuretic. Stops bleeding. (**Cautions!** Seek medical advice for blood in the urine or other bleeding disorders, including the onset of sudden heavy menses. Contains saponins, which should not be used on broken skin, as they can dissolve red blood cells.)

Hyssop (*Hyssopus officinalis*). The flowers are a relaxing expectorant and peripheral vasodilator; used for respiratory ills and flu. Often suggested for children. (**Caution!** Stick to recommended doses and short-term use. In large doses, the essential oil could cause convulsions.)

Irish moss (*Chondrus crispus*). This is actually a seaweed or red alga. A demulcent, expectorant, nutritive, and emulsifier. Prevents vomiting.

Jewelweed (*Impatiens pallida* [yellow flowers] or *I. capensis* [orange flowers]; also called touch-me-not). This is a common, very tall wildflower with watery stems. The fruits explode if touched, which is where the touch-me-not name comes from. (Children are much entertained by this harmless trait.) The juice from the stems is commonly used externally to treat poison ivy and insect bites and stings. Some say it can prevent poison ivy if applied before contact with the plant.

Jimsonweed (*Datura stramonium;* also called Jamestown weed or thorn apple). The aerial parts are both sedating and stimulating to the central nervous system. A bronchial and visceral antispasmodic. (**Cautions!** Restricted in some countries. High doses may cause depression, depressed cerebral or respiratory function, tachycardia, and even coma. Especially avoid in pregnancy, with glaucoma, or with other depressants. Many herbals suggest avoiding this one altogether, but especially without expert medical advice.)

Juniper (*Juniperus communis*). The berries are used for their potent diuretic, digestive, and antirheumatic actions and in making gin. Some commercially prepared water pills (to reduce bloating) contain juniper oil. (**Cautions!** Avoid in pregnancy [possible link with miscarriage] or with kidney trouble. Long-term use may damage the kidneys. Do not eat the berries, which may deliver too high a dose of the oil.)

Kelp (*Fucus vesiculosus;* also called bladder wrack, black tang, or rockweed; *Laminaria longicruris*). A common seaweed in the Atlantic Ocean and other areas. A metabolic stimulant, nutritive, and thyroid restorative. Contains iodine. An adaptogen, used for various thyroid ills, though best used with the advice of a medical practitioner. (**Caution!** Harvesting needs to be done in uncontaminated areas. Beware of metal pollutants. Seek a reputable source.)

Lady's-mantle (*Alchemilla vulgaris;* also called lion's foot). The flowers are used as an astringent, digestive, and anti-inflammatory and to regulate the menses. Suggested for gynecological ills but also a uterine stimulant. (**Caution!** Avoid in pregnancy.)

Lady's slipper (*Cypripedium pubescens;* also called American valerian). A protected species in some regions; not to be harvested in the wild. The rhizome has sedative actions, as the name American valerian suggests. An antispasmodic and nervine.

Lavender (*Lavandula officinalis*). The flowers are a relaxant, antispasmodic, circulatory stimulant, diuretic, nerve tonic, and uterine stimulant. The essential oil is sometimes suggested for external application against headaches or rheumatic ills. (**Caution!** Avoid in pregnancy.)

Lemon balm (*Melissa officinalis;* also called bee balm, balm, or honey plant). Just the leaves are used as a sedative, antidepressant, digestive, and antispasmodic. Antiviral and antibacterial. The U.S. Food and Drug Administration says it's "generally recognized as safe." (**Caution!** Lemon balm has been linked with inhibiting some thyroid hormones, so it should be avoided or monitored by a doctor for anyone with Graves' disease or other thyroid difficulties.)

Lemon verbena (*Aloysia triphylla*). Mainly used as an aromatic, for the bath, and as a strewing herb.

Licorice (*Glycyrrhiza glabra* or, in China, *G. uralensis* [gan cao]). The roots and stolons are used. Considered a blood detoxifier by some. An expectorant and anti-inflammatory. Soothes gastric membranes and lowers blood cholesterol. The U.S. Food and Drug Administration says it's "generally recognized as safe." Most licorice candies do not contain the true herb. (**Cautions!** Avoid in hypertension or with high blood pressure, glaucoma, heart conditions, or kidney disease. Avoid in combination with digitalis, digoxin-based drugs, or asthma medicines. Can cause fluid retention. Can affect blood potassium. Contains saponins, which should not be used on broken skin, as they can dissolve red blood cells.)

Liferoot (*Senecio aureus;* also called golden groundsel or squaw-weed). Do not confuse with squaw vine (*Mitchella repens*). This root is a uterine relaxant and stimulant to the gravid uterus; soothing to the nervous system. (**Caution!** Avoid in pregnancy.)

Lime. See Linden.

Linden (*Tilia europaea;* also called lime). The flowers are used. A nervine with sedating actions; relaxes and helps heal blood vessels; may help prevent arteriosclerosis. A diuretic and peripheral vasodilator (increasing blood supply to the tissues). Sometimes suggested for fever.

Linseed (*Linum usitatissimum;* also called flaxseed). The seed is used as a laxative, expectorant, and local antiseptic. Another form, the mountain flax (*L. catharticum*), is a more potent laxative, as its Latin name suggests, and is sometimes used instead of senna. If you use it, be wary of its purgative powers. (**Cautions!** Do not use artists' or hardware store versions of linseed oil for internal or medicinal uses. Deteriorates rapidly. Seeds contain prussic acid, which is toxic in very high doses.)

Lobelia (*Lobelia inflata;* also called pukeweed or Indian tobacco). The aerial parts are used as an expectorant, emetic, and antispasmodic. (**Cautions!** This is a controlled substance in some countries. Can cause difficulty breathing. Contains a nicotinelike alkaloid. Emetic in large doses, as the common name pukeweed denotes. Use in small doses and seek expert advice.)

Lovage (*Levisticum officinale*). The root is a digestive, antispasmodic, expectorant, diuretic, and anticatarrhal. Sometimes the seeds are used.

Maidenhair fern (*Adiantum pedatum*). Used for urinary stones, stitches (sharp pains) in the side, respiratory ills, hair growth, and swelling.

Maidenhair tree. See Ginkgo.

Mallow (*Malva sylvestris,* common mallow; *M. crispa,* French mallow). *M. sylvestris* is commonly used in poultices for wounds. Parkinson lists French mallow as a potherb. See also Marshmallow.

Marigold. See Calendula.

Marjoram (*Origanum marjorana*). The leaves and essential oil are sometimes used medicinally to promote the menses or as an antispasmodic.

Marshmallow (*Althaea officinalis*). The flowers are used as an expectorant, the leaves for bronchial or urinary disorders. The roots are a demulcent, expectorant, and diuretic and are used externally on wounds or burns. Both leaves and roots are mucilaginous.

Meadowsweet (*Filipendula ulmaria; Spiraea ulmaria,* also called queen of the meadow or bridewort; *S. latifolia*). The dried flowers and leaves are used as a diuretic, anti-inflammatory, and astringent and to soothe gastric mucosa. Commonly used as a strewing herb. Some herbalists consider it a uterine stimulant. (**Cautions!** Contains salicin, an aspirinlike component. Pregnant women and children under 16 should not take herbs containing salicin because of the risks associated with aspirin and birth defects or Reye's syndrome. Those with ulcers or gastritis should seek medical advice before using it.)

Milk thistle (*Carduus marianus*). The seeds are used to stimulate bile flow and may help protect the liver from degenerative diseases, including alcoholism. (**Caution!** Seek a doctor's advice about liver problems.)

Motherwort (*Leonurus cardiaca*). A member of the Labiatae family. Culpeper said it makes "women joyful mothers of children" and settles their wombs. Modern research suggests it's more apt to prevent motherhood than promote it. It's a uterine stimulant and trigger to the menses but might aid in expelling the afterbirth. The Greeks and Romans used it for heart palpitations, and in Japan it's thought to promote longevity. A nerve tonic and sedative, motherwort infusions (leaves and flowers) are sometimes used for menstrual problems, menopausal symptoms, and after childbirth. (**Cautions!** Do not use if pregnant, except possibly at full term, with the advice of your health practitioner, as a uterine stimulant. May have an anticlotting effect on the blood; seek medical advice regarding heart conditions and its use.)

Mugwort (*Artemisia vulgaris; A. absinthium,* wormwood). An aromatic moth repellent. Named for Artemis, Greek goddess of the moon, the hunt, and chastity. Called the oldest of the worts, mugwort grows wild from Nova Scotia to Michigan. True to Artemis, who loved the chase, mugwort was thought to protect travelers from fatigue, lightning, sunstroke, the evil eye, plague, and wild beasts. Placed under a horse's saddle, it refreshed the steed. Walkers stuffed it in their shoes. The druids of Devon and Cornwall, England, used it to lure the sun's warmth back to earth. American Indians put a leaf in one nostril to cure headaches. The Chinese make a moxibustion cone of mugwort and burn it at the feet of a pregnant woman in hopes of preventing a breech birth. Nicholas Culpeper advised using mugwort "for a good time" or using the smoke of it under a child's bed "to make him merry and take away annox [anxiety]." Mugwort leaves and flowers are sometimes infused and taken for menopausal symptoms or menstrual pain.

The aerial parts of wormwood (also infused, weakly) are used against worms and parasites, for hepatitis and jaundice, and for poor digestion. Wormwood is a common strewing herb and is burned as incense for its aroma. Both species are bitter digestives and uterine stimulants. (**Caution!** Avoid during pregnancy and while nursing. May cause fetal abnormalities if used during pregnancy.)

Mulberry (*Morus nigra* or *M. alba*). The berries may be used as a laxative. The leaves are antibacterial and may be used as an expectorant. The root bark may be used as a sedative and diuretic and can lower blood pressure. Rarely used today. (**Caution!** Avoid with diarrhea.)

Mullein. See Great mullein.

Mustard (*Sinapis alba*, yellow or white mustard; *Brassica nigra*, black mustard; *B. juncea*, brown mustard). The seeds of all three types are commonly used medicinally, especially in heat-producing plasters or poultices. (**Cautions!** Direct body contact can cause blistering; a layer of cheesecloth and careful attention are recommended. In large quantities or prolonged use, mustard can depress thyroid function. Internal use can irritate the stomach; those with ulcers may want to avoid it.)

Myrrh (*Commiphora molmol*). The resin is used as an antiseptic, astringent, antifungal agent, and expectorant. A uterine stimulant. Considered by some to be an immune stimulant. (**Caution!** Avoid if pregnant.)

Nettle (*Urtica dioica* or *U. urens*; also called stinging nettle). The aerial parts are generally used, although the roots are sometimes decocted for hair rinses. A nutritive, diuretic, astringent, and circulatory stimulant. Promotes lactation. (**Cautions!** Lowers blood sugar levels. Large doses can irritate the stomach, deplete minerals, and lead to dehydration.)

Nutmeg (*Myristica fragrans*). The powdered fruit is an antispasmodic, anti-inflammatory, digestive, and gastric stimulant. Prevents vomiting and promotes appetite. Mace, the outer part of the fruit, was sometimes used in rheumatism ointments. (**Caution!** Very large doses of nutmeg could be overly stimulating to the central nervous system, causing convulsions or heart palpitations.)

Oats (*Avena sativa*). The whole oat plant, harvested when the seeds are ripe, is called *oat straw*. *Oat bran* and *oatmeal* are derivative forms and somewhat less active, though effective in reducing blood cholesterol. Oat straw, the usual medicinal, is considered restorative to the nervous system. (**Caution!** Some people are sensitive to the gluten in oats.)

Onion. See Alliums.

Parsley (*Petroselinum crispum, P. sativum,* or *Carum petroselinium*). The aerial parts are a strong diuretic, digestive, antispasmodic, and uterine stimulant. (**Caution!** Avoid the seeds or heavy consumption of the herb, as in a parsley pesto, during pregnancy.)

Passionflower (*Passiflora incarnata*). The leaves have an antispasmodic effect and some sedative and hypnotic properties. May reduce pain or promote sleep. (**Caution!** Avoid in large doses in pregnancy.)

Peppermint (*Mentha × piperita*). Peppermint is really a hybrid of water mint and spearmint. The aerial parts are used as an antispasmodic, peripheral vasodilator, and analgesic. Used for fever and to reduce morning sickness. Reduces lactation. The U.S. Food and Drug Administration says it's "generally recognized as safe." (**Cautions!** Do not give any of the mints directly to babies. Do not use if breast-feeding. For short-term use [not more than a week], especially with children; can irritate mucous linings if inhaled or consumed over a long period. Pure menthol is toxic; avoid ingesting peppermint oil.)

Peruvian bark (*Cinchona succirubra* or *C. officinalis;* also called cinchona). A bitter digestive and uterine stimulant. Sometimes suggested for drunkenness. (**Cautions!** Avoid if pregnant. For short-term use only. Incompatible with salicylates. Restricted in some countries, such as Great Britain.)

Plantain (*Plantago major;* also called greater plantain or rat's tail). A common roadside weed. Plantain leaves are generally used externally for poultices and to relieve insect bites and stings. Sometimes used internally for gastric or urinary ills. A demulcent, astringent, expectorant, and diuretic. Note: *P. major* is not related to the banana-like plantain (*Musa paradisiaca*).

Pleurisy root (*Asclepias tuberosa;* also called whiteroot, butterfly weed, orange milkweed, or windroot). An expectorant and vasodilator. Reputed to be soothing to the respiratory system.

Poplar (*Populus tremuloides;* also called quaking aspen or white poplar). The dried bark contains salicin, an aspirinlike component. Used as a digestive, diuretic, and astringent. (**Cautions!** Pregnant women and children under 16 should not take herbs containing salicin because of the risks associated with aspirin and birth defects or Reye's syndrome.)

Prickly ash (*Zanthoxylum americanum,* also called toothache tree; *Z. clavaherculis*). The bark and berries are sometimes used as a circulatory stimulant or locally as a counterirritant.

Primrose. See Cowslip.

Pukeweed. See Lobelia.

Purple coneflower. See Echinacea.

Purslane (*Portulaca oleracea*). A potherb (now considered a weed by many) commonly grown in kitchen gardens and used in salads or for a quick thirst quencher. Purslane also was used internally for jaundice and applied externally for toothache or sore eyes.

Raspberry (*Rubus idaeus*). The leaves are usually used. The berries are sometimes recommended for rheumatic disorders or indigestion. The common North American raspberry, *R. strigosus*, is sometimes substituted for *R. idaeus*. Provides toning action to the gravid uterus and sometimes suggested for late pregnancy (last trimester). Locally astringent and sometimes used as a gargle. (**Caution!** Avoid high doses in the first six months of pregnancy, as it may act as a uterine stimulant.)

Red clover (*Trifolium pratense*; also called three-leaved grass, purple clover, or trefoil). The flowers are a diuretic, expectorant, antispasmodic, and anti-inflammatory, with possible estrogenic effects. Has been used experimentally with breast, ovarian, and lymphatic cancers. Sometimes suggested for topical skin inflammations or arthritis pain. The U.S. Food and Drug Administration says it's "generally recognized as safe."

Rheumatism root. See Wild yam.

Rhubarb (*Rheum palmatum*). The root is used medicinally. (The cooking version, made into pies and other dishes, is generally *R. rhabarbarum*, a more recent cultivar.) A powerful purgative, laxative, digestive, and astringent; antibacterial. (**Cautions!** Too strong for children. The leaves are toxic. Avoid in pregnancy. The root contains calcium oxalate and is best avoided in arthritic conditions or gout.)

Rose — rose hips (*Rosa canina*; also called dog rose or brier rose). High in vitamin C, rose hips are used as an antidepressant, antispasmodic, astringent, sedative, digestive, expectorant, anti-inflammatory, and antibacterial and antiviral agent. Sometimes suggested for colds, respiratory infections, or gastric distress. Various teas contain rose hips. The Chinese use *R. rugosa* flowers as an energy stimulant and blood tonic. *R. damascena* (damask rose) flowers are distilled into the Bulgarian rose oil often used in expensive perfumes and also used medicinally as an antidepressant and sedative. (**Cautions!** Do not substitute hybrid or garden roses for those listed here. Rose oil is generally considered nontoxic but should be used internally only with expert advice. Also, rose oil is frequently adulterated and difficult to find in its pure — and expensive — form.)

Rosemary (*Rosmarinus officinalis*). The aerial parts are used as an antispasmodic, relaxant, stimulant to peripheral circulation, and nervine. Possibly a cardiac tonic. The essential oil is sometimes suggested for topical use for rheumatic ills, as an analgesic, and as a hair tonic. Reputed to restore color to brown hair. (**Cautions!** Avoid in medicinal doses if pregnant, but OK for cooking in normal quantities. Do not ingest the oil. Large quantities of rosemary can cause gastric or kidney distress or cramping.)

Rue (*Ruta graveolens;* also called herb of grace). The leaves are a uterine and circulatory stimulant, expectorant, and emetic. (**Cautions!** Avoid in pregnancy because of its emetic properties. Use low doses even if not pregnant for the same reason. Best if used with expert advice.)

Sage (*Salvia officinalis;* also called red sage). The leaves are reputed to enhance longevity. Antibiotic, astringent, antiseptic, and antispasmodic actions. Reduces blood sugar. Relaxes peripheral blood vessels. Contains estrogenic substances. (**Cautions!** Avoid medicinal doses if pregnant. Normal cooking quantities are considered OK in pregnancy. Avoid if epileptic because its thujone can trigger fits. Sage oil may be toxic. Some people report mouth or lip troubles in reaction to sage tea, but others find it an ideal gargle or mouthwash. Blood sugar and blood vessel effects should be monitored by medical experts. Reduces lactation, so avoid if breast-feeding.) See also Clary.

Saint Johnswort (*Hypericum perforatum*). A yellow-flowered herb named for St. John the Baptist, whose feast day is June 24, when the plant is in bloom. The Greek *hyper,* "above," and *eikon,* "picture," refer to the custom of hanging the herb over images to ward off evil. It also decorated cottage windows and doorways as protection against lightning. There were those who claimed that if you cut it after sunset, a fairy horse would carry you off until daybreak.

Saint Johnswort was believed to cure bed-wetting, to protect against hydrophobia and madness, and to promote healthy crops. Saint Johnswort was used on battlefields for more than 2,000 years and was used extensively during the American Civil War. Brazilians also used it for snakebite. Today Saint Johnswort goes into Hypericin, an experimental AIDS drug being researched in the United States, Germany, and the former Soviet Union. An ointment of the herb is prescribed for skin complaints and burns. An infusion of the flowers is used for chest complaints and depression and as a gargle, astringent, nervine, and expectorant. (**Caution!** Can cause skin problems if taken internally and the skin is exposed to the sun.)

Sarsaparilla (*Smilax* spp.). The root is used as a circulatory stimulant and has some testosteronal properties. Sometimes suggested for rheumatic ills. Once commonly an ingredient in soft drinks.

Sassafras (*Sassafras albidum;* also called cinnamonwood or ague tree). The root and bark were commonly used before modern-day cautions were known. (**Cautions!** Sassafras has been linked with cancer. Do not ingest! The volatile oil contains safrole, which is toxic to the nervous system and blood.)

Saw palmetto (*Serenoa serrulata* or *Sabal serrulata*). The berries are a diuretic, anticatarrhal, and urinary antiseptic. Sometimes suggested for male reproductive functions or for reducing an enlarged prostate. (**Cautions!** Obtain expert medical advice about prostate troubles or blood in the urine. Saw palmetto can interact unfavorably with traditional prostate medicines. Can influence screening tests for prostate cancer and give a misleading reading. Seek the oil-based extracts and look for pure, reputable sources.)

Self-heal (*Prunella vulgaris;* also called xia ku cao or carpenter's herb). The aerial parts and flower spikes are an antioxidant, antibacterial agent, and diuretic. Reduces blood pressure. By the doctrine of signatures, considered useful for throat ailments. Traditionally used for headaches. In China, used against fever and liver and kidney disorders. (**Caution!** Avoid if you have low blood pressure.)

Shepherd's purse (*Capsella bursa-pastoris;* also called mother's-heart). Used primarily as a styptic to stop bleeding, the aerial parts of shepherd's purse are also a circulatory and uterine stimulant, astringent, and urinary antiseptic. Reduces blood pressure. (**Cautions!** Avoid in pregnancy, except possibly during labor and under medical advice. Consult medical experts about any bleeding disorder or blood in the urine. Avoid if low blood pressure is a problem.)

Skullcap (*Scutellaria laterifolia* or *S. galericulata*). The dried aerial parts are an antispasmodic, relaxing to the nervous system. May help treat epileptic symptoms. (**Caution!** Germander, which has been suggested to be toxic to the liver, is occasionally sold as skullcap. Be certain of your source.)

Skunk cabbage (*Symplocarpus foetidus;* also called meadow cabbage). The roots and rhizomes are used much like onions, as an expectorant and antispasmodic. Native Americans considered it a contraceptive. (**Caution!** Avoid if pregnant or trying to conceive.)

Slippery elm (*Ulmus rubra;* also called red elm or moose elm). The inner bark is used for its demulcent and emollient properties. Somewhat nutritive. Often used in cough drops or throat lozenges. Considered soothing to mucous membranes.

Soapbark (*Quillaja saponaria*). The bark is a sudsing agent and anti-inflammatory. (**Cautions!** For external use only. Contains saponins, which should not be used on broken skin, as they can dissolve red blood cells.)

Soapwort (*Saponaria officinalis*). The roots are used for soap or shampoo. Native Americans used it to stun fish in a pool. Can be used topically against itchy skin and rheumatism. (**Cautions!** For external use only. Contains saponins, which should not be used on broken skin, as they can dissolve red blood cells.)

Southernwood (*Artemisia abrotanum;* also called lad's-love or old man). The aerial parts are a uterine stimulant and digestive; once suggested for intestinal worms, as a hair rinse, or, most commonly, as a strewing herb. (**Caution!** Avoid if pregnant.)

Squawroot. See Black cohosh and Blue cohosh.

Stickwort. See Agrimony.

Sweet cicely (*Myrrhis odorata* or *Osmorhiza* spp.). Little known or used today. (**Caution!** Poison hemlock [*Conium maculatum*] is an herbal look-alike, so use extreme care in identifying these plants.)

Sweet sumac (*Rhus aromatic*). The bark of the root is an astringent, antidiabetic agent, and diuretic. (**Caution!** Diabetics should seek expert advice about its possible use.)

Sweet violet (*Viola odorata*). The aerial parts are an expectorant, diuretic, and anti-inflammatory; some say they have antitumor properties. (**Caution!** Because of the saponins in sweet violet, avoid very high doses, which could cause vomiting or nausea.) See also Heartsease.

Tansy (*Tanacetum vulgare;* also called gold buttons). Generally regarded as a strewing herb now, although once used in tansy cakes and other ceremonial recipes and in amulets worn against worms. (**Cautions!** Tansy is a narcotic and can cause miscarriage or fetal damage in high doses. Avoid its internal use. Even external use may cause contact dermatitis.)

Tea (*Camellia sinensis*). There are many varieties of tea leaves and other tea ingredients, and each has its own properties and applications. The three main types are *green teas,* which are rich in fluoride and may enhance the immune system and help prevent certain cancers; *oolong teas,* which are partly fermented and often used to reduce blood cholesterol and lower blood pressure; and *black teas,* which are fully fermented, highly astringent, and good for diarrhea. (**Cautions!** All three types contain caffeine, so they should be used in moderation by pregnant or nursing mothers, anyone with an irregular heartbeat or other heart condition, and anyone with stomach troubles.)

Tea tree oil (*Melaleuca alternifolia;* also called ti tree oil). This essential oil is used externally as a powerful antibacterial agent. (**Caution!** Do not ingest.)

Thyme (*Thymus vulgaris,* also called common thyme; *T. serpyllum,* also called wild thyme). The aerial parts are a uterine stimulant, antiseptic, expectorant, diuretic, antispasmodic, antibiotic, and astringent. The U.S. Food and Drug Administration says it's "generally recognized as safe." (**Cautions!** Avoid therapeutic doses in pregnancy [cooking uses OK]. Thyme oil can irritate mucous membranes.)

Turmeric (*Curcuma longa*). The powdered rootstock of the plant is used medicinally, ceremonially, and as a dye. An antioxidant. Reduces blood cholesterol. An anti-inflammatory, sometimes used for rheumatic disorders. May protect the stomach lining and help prevent ulcers. Being studied for its anticancer properties, especially with smokers. (**Cautions!** High doses can irritate the stomach. Should not be given in therapeutic doses to young children. May hamper conception, but studies are inconclusive.)

Unicorn root, false. See False unicorn root.

Valerian (*Valeriana officinalis;* also called all-heal or garden heliotrope). Do not confuse this plant with the common red American valerian (*Centranthus ruber*), which does not share its medicinal properties. The fresh or dried root is used, often in candy, tobacco products, baked goods, and beverages and sometimes in cat toys. Available in capsules. Once used to treat epilepsy and to bring on the menses; later used as a tranquilizer, diuretic, expectorant, antispasmodic, and sleep aid, as well as to counter fatigue. The U.S. Food and Drug Administration says it's "generally recognized as safe." (**Cautions!** An overdose may cause headache, vomiting, delusions, muscle spasms, dizziness, or depression. Can lead to overexcitement. Start any treatment with small doses. Never boil. Not only do cats crave the smell, but rats like it as well. The roots are sometimes used for rat trap bait.)

Vervain (*Verbena officinalis;* also called verbena or blue vervain). The aerial parts are a uterine stimulant, nervine, sedative, and liver restorative. Promotes lactation. (**Caution!** Avoid in pregnancy.)

Violet. See Sweet violet and Heartsease.

White willow (*Salix alba;* also called European willow). The bark contains salicin and has pain-relieving properties. May help prevent heart attack, stroke, and migraine. An antirheumatic, anti-inflammatory, analgesic, antiseptic, astringent, and digestive. (**Cautions!** Pregnant women and children under 16 should not take herbs containing salicin because of the risks associated with aspirin and birth defects or Reye's syndrome.)

Wild yam (*Dioscorea villosa;* also called rheumatism root, colicroot, yam, Mexican wild yam; *D. quaternata*). The rhizome is an antispasmodic, peripheral vasodilator, and anti-inflammatory. Contains hormonal substances resembling progesterone. (**Cautions!** Avoid in pregnancy, particularly in high doses, except possibly during labor and with expert advice. Contains saponins, which should not be used on broken skin, as they can dissolve red blood cells.)

Willow. See White willow.

Wintergreen (*Gaultheria procumbens;* also called checkerberry or teaberry). The leaves and aerial stems are an anti-inflammatory and diuretic. Contains salicins. (**Cautions!** Avoid oil of wintergreen, generally derived from a species of birch, which can be toxic; do not ingest. Pregnant women and children under 16 should not take herbs containing salicin because of the risks associated with aspirin and birth defects or Reye's syndrome.)

Witch hazel (*Hamamelis virginiana*). The bark or leaves are decocted for their astringent actions. (**Caution!** Use externally.)

Wood betony (*Betonica officinalis* or *Stachys betonica*). The aerial parts are used most often, although the roots were once used as a liver tonic and laxative.

A tannin, bitter stimulant to digestion, uterine stimulant, and astringent. (**Cautions!** Large doses are emetic and cathartic. Best not to use for children. Avoid in pregnancy.)

Wormwood. See Mugwort.

Yam. See Wild yam.

Yarrow (*Achillea millefolium;* also called woundwort). Achilles' secret against bleeding. Woundwort was used to stanch the flow of blood during the Battle of Troy as well as in the American Civil War. Folklore valued it for self-esteem and love charms, to conjure the Devil, and against heartache and insomnia. American Indians used it to stay baldness, and in India it's a fever remedy. Brought to weddings, it's supposed to ensure seven years of love, but any woman caught gathering it may be labeled a witch. An infusion of the flowers or aerial parts is used for colds and flu and for digestive and urinary problems. A uterine stimulant. (**Cautions!** Avoid in pregnancy. Some people experience skin rashes or photosensitivity from yarrow.)

Yellow dock (*Rumex crispus;* also called curly dock or narrow-leaved dock). The root is used as a cleansing laxative and to promote bile.

A Glossary of Terms

Aerial parts. The aboveground parts of a plant — notably, the leaves, stems, and flowers.

Ague. An acute fever or fit of alternating chills and heat.

Alkaloid. A highly active plant constituent containing nitrogen and often toxic in high doses. Caffeine and nicotine are alkaloids; others occur in comfrey, Saint Johnswort, and wood betony. (See Appendix I for cautions about the potential dangers of these and other ingredients.)

Alum. A powdered form of a topical astringent or styptic, available in pharmacies and health food stores; any of various double sulfates of a trivalent metal that can be used medicinally.

Amulet. A small bag, object, or charm worn to protect the wearer from ill health or other evil. Garlic cloves, camphor, and other remedies were strung on necklaces or placed in small bags and worn against disease.

Analgesic. Easing pain. Mulberry branches and twigs have natural analgesic properties.

Anaphrodisiac. Decreasing sexual desire. Some soporific herbs, such as hops, are considered anaphrodisiac.

Anemia. Iron deficiency in the blood or, sometimes, lack of vitamin B_{12}, possibly causing fatigue, poor resistance to infection, and pallor. Women, especially those with heavy menses, are particularly prone to iron-poor anemia.

Anesthetic. Numbing sensation; reducing the feeling of pain.

Antibacterial. Destroying bacteria. Garlic and rhubarb are antibacterial.

Antibiotic. Destroying bacteria (as in prescription drugs for earaches or strep throat). Burdock root and purple coneflower exhibit antibiotic actions.

Antihistamine. Neutralizing histamine in allergies and colds.

Antioxidant. Inhibiting oxidation; a protective nutrient to block the chemical reactions by which many toxins (such as air pollution) cause harm to the human body. Vitamins C and E are antioxidant.

Antiscorbutic. Preventing or treating scurvy. Vinegar, citrus fruits, and other sources of vitamin C are antiscorbutic.

Antiseptic. Preventing putrefaction. All volatile oils are antiseptic to some degree, although most are not so strong as to demonstrate the property on contact. The higher the level of tannin in an herb, the stronger its antiseptic properties.

Antispasmodic. Preventing or relieving cramps and spasms. Ginger is antispasmodic.

Antiviral. Destroying or reducing viral growth and infections. Lemon balm has antiviral actions.

Aperient. A mild laxative.

Aphrodisiac. Increasing sexual desire. From Aphrodite, the Greek goddess of love.

Apothecary. A storehouse of medicinals; a pharmacist.

Aromatic. A particularly fragrant plant or substance; sometimes used medicinally, as in aromatherapy.

Astringent. Contracting to the skin; reducing secretions. Goldenseal and witch hazel are naturally astringent.

Bile. A bitter, alkaline secretion of the liver that aids digestion, chiefly by saponifying fats.

Bilious attack. Usually a mislabeling of indigestion (acid stomach) or heartburn; literally, too much bile.

Bitter. A digestive or tonic herb such as dandelion, rosemary, or burdock root. Bitters stimulate the appetite, increase digestive juices, and increase the flow of bile. Wormwood and mugwort are both bitter digestive tonics (and uterine stimulants); see Appendix I for cautions.

Blister. To raise a blister on the skin.

Bruise. To crush or beat, as a spice in a mortar and pestle.

Carcinogen. A cancer-producing agent.

Carminative. Easing digestive gas, abdominal cramps, and flatulence. Fennel, cardamom, cinnamon, ginger, parsley, peppermint, thyme, celery, hyssop, and motherwort are carminative.

Castile soap. A fine soap originally from Castile, Spain, made of olive oil and soda; available in hard or liquid form from health food stores and some pharmacies.

Catarrh. Excessive mucus secretions in the respiratory system, often accompanied by wheezing, coughing, or other cold symptoms.

Catarrhal. Reducing mucus and catarrh.

Chin stay. A compress applied to the chin area.

Citric acid. The powdered crystalline acid derived from the fermentation of carbohydrates or from lemon, lime, or pineapple juice; available from pharmacies and health food stores.

Clister. An enema; a remedy administered to the rectum for cleansing or to offer nourishment when other means fail. Also clyster or glyster.

Cold condition. Chills, fatigue, poor circulation, sharp pains, frequent passing of urine, and thirst for hot drinks.

Colic. Pains in the abdomen, cramps; often applied to babies with digestive distress. Sometimes called grippe or grip.

Comfit. A sweetmeat, such as caraway seeds sugared and preserved.

Compress. Layers of flannel or other cloth soaked in water or an herbal infusion or decoction and then applied warm or cold to the body. A lavender compress might be applied to the temples for headache pain, for example.

Concoct. To boil together or prepare by mixing; to invent, devise, or contrive.

Constipation. Sluggish or infrequent bowel movements; sometimes hard stools.

Cordial. An invigorating drink, generally alcoholic.

Costive, costiveness. Constipated, constipation.

Cradle cap. A child's dermatitis, showing yellowish or brownish flakes or lesions on the scalp.

Dandruff. Scaling or flaking of the top layers of the scalp.

Decoct. To extract the flavor by boiling; to concentrate or boil down. From the Latin *de* (down) and *coquere* (to cook). Usually an herb is mixed with water, boiled or simmered for 10 to 20 minutes, and then strained and used in liquid form.

Demulcent. Soothing to the mucous membranes or other tissues. Mullein is demulcent, as is aloe vera.

Deobstruent. Removing obstructions.

Diaphoretic. Promoting sweating or perspiration. Ginger is diaphoretic.

Diarrhea. Frequent and very liquid stools, which, if severe or prolonged, can lead to dehydration, especially in young children; sometimes called "summer complaint."

Diuretic. Increasing the production of urine. Burdock leaves, asparagus, parsley, dandelion leaves, celery, birch, broom, horsetail, juniper, and coffee are diuretic.

Doctrine of signatures. The theory that symptoms (or signatures) of an illness correspond to the shape or color of a plant that can be used to cure the illness. For example, the flower heads of poppies, shaped like a skull, would be good for diseases of the head; walnuts, which look like the brain, would be brain food; and red rose petals would be good for the blood. Sometimes called law of signatures.

Drachm. Three scruples, 60 grains, or ⅛ ounce. Also dram or drachma.

Dropsy. The pathological accumulation of diluted lymph in body tissues; bloating and continual thirst.

Dysentery. Severe diarrhea, sometimes bloody or containing mucus. Dysentery can be either a parasitic or a bacterial infection.

Dyspepsia. A digestive distress, possibly exhibiting nausea or heartburn, bloating, belching, gassiness, and abdominal pain, sometimes with vomiting. May be caused by an excess of rich foods or alcohol. Dyspepsia bread is a digestive bread usually made with bran, or "unbolted" wheat flour.

Eczema. A condition that involves itchy, very dry, or inflamed skin.

Elixir. A sweetened, aromatic drink usually containing alcohol, water, and various medicinals. Sometimes used to mean a cure-all.

Embrocation. A liniment.

Emetic. Causing nausea and vomiting.

Emollient. Soothing to the skin; healing of irritations.

Enema. A cleansing or nutritive treatment applied through the rectum, clearing it of feces.

Enuresis. Involuntary urination; bed-wetting.

Episiotomy. A surgical incision of the perineum during childbirth; sometimes performed to facilitate delivery and avoid tearing.

Epsom salts. Hydrated magnesium sulfate, sometimes used as a remedy for constipation and other ills; a cathartic. The name comes from Epsom, England.

Essential oil. A volatile oil or scented plant oil, usually having the characteristic odor or flavor of the plant, distilled by steam to the basic essence, which contains active components.

Exfoliant. Something that causes the skin to cast off dry flakes of dead skin. Mashed apple or a paste of oats or couscous can be used as an exfoliant to rejuvenate skin.

Expectorant. Promoting the expulsion of mucus, such as an expectorant cough syrup helping to expel phlegm from the lungs. White horehound is an expectorant often used in cough drops; plantain is another expectorant.

Falling down of the fundament. Uterine prolapse in women or scrotal hernia in men; also a protrusion of part of the rectum (hemorrhoids, or piles).

Flatulence. Gas in the stomach or bowels, sometimes causing pain or cramping. Certain foods, such as beans, onions, and eggs, can promote flatulence, especially in those prone to the condition.

Flooding. Uterine hemorrhage or very heavy period.

Flu. Influenza.

Flux. Diarrhea.

Fomentation. A warm, moist medicinal compress or poultice.

Gallipot. A small, glazed earthenware jar for medicinals.

Gill. A unit of measure equaling four fluid ounces.

Glycerol. A syrupy, sweet yellowish liquid used as a solvent for some herbal preparations — for instance, to replace alcohol as the base of a tincture. Also glycerin(e).

Glycoside. An organic compound that produces sugars and related substances on hydrolysis; occurs, for instance, in soapwort, dock, mullein, and licorice. From glycose, a variant of glucose, which is used in confectionary and alcoholic fermentation.

Gravel. Urinary or kidney stones, obstructions, or crystals; pain in passing urine.

Grippe. See Colic.

Gruel. A watery porridge.

Halitosis. Bad breath; sometimes caused by decaying teeth or gums or by constipation.

Hartshorn. A substance obtained by rasping the antlers of a stag. Used as a source of ammonia or smelling salts. Also hart's horn.

Heat ring. A ring of ceramic or other porous, nonflammable material placed over a warm light bulb to disseminate an aromatic, volatile oil that has been dripped onto it.

Hemorrhoids. Varicose veins in the rectum, sometimes associated with constipation or pregnancy. Also called piles.

Homeopathy. Theory of treatment in which a small amount of a substance that causes an illness is given to stimulate the body's immune reaction.

Hysterectomy. The surgical removal of the uterus, or womb.

Immunity. Resistance to disease.

Impotence. A male's inability to achieve or complete sexual intercourse.

Incontinence. Lack of urinary control; involuntary urination (see Enuresis).

Incubation period. The time between the contraction of an illness and the appearance of symptoms.

Infertility. The inability to conceive and reproduce.

Influenza. A viral infection, often in epidemics, characterized by respiratory distress, fever, headache, and muscle aches. Incubation period is commonly two to four days. Also called flu.

Infuse. To steep or soak without boiling in order to extract soluble elements or active principles; to pour. An infusion is generally considered stronger than a tea.

Insomnia. Sleeplessness; the inability to remain asleep for normal periods of time.

Jaundice. A yellowish color to the skin caused by excessive bile. Premature babies are prone to jaundice because of insufficiently developed livers.

Jigger. A measure of alcohol, usually containing 1½ ounces.

Kitchen garden. Distinguished from an orchard or "falling garden," pleasure garden of ornamentals, or parlor garden of formal design, a kitchen garden or woman's cottage garden was the source of medicinals, strewing herbs, and practical potherbs, generally located for easy access near the kitchen.

Lactation. The production of milk by the mammary glands for breast-feeding the young.

Laryngitis. An inflammation of the voice box, or larynx.

Larynx. The voice box.

Laxative. Promoting bowel movements. Castor oil is laxative.

Leukorrhea. A vaginal discharge. Sometimes referred to as the "whites." Also leucorrhea.

Libido. Sexual drive or energy.

Liniment. A medicinal fluid rubbed into the skin as a local anesthetic or counterirritant. Herb extracts in liniments, such as cayenne pepper, ginger, or mustard, may be used to increase circulation or heat; others, such as mints, are cooling.

Loaf sugar. Sugar refined and molded into a loaf shape.

Looseness. Diarrhea.

Macerate. To make soft, usually by steeping in a liquid; to separate into constituents by soaking.

Mastitis. An inflammation of the breast or milk ducts, especially during breast-feeding and weaning.

Menarche. The first menstrual period.

Menopause. The time around the last menstrual period.

Menses. Menstrual discharge.

Migraine. A severe, throbbing headache, sometimes temporarily affecting vision or causing nausea or vomiting. Women are more prone to migraines than men. The menses can trigger them, as can certain foods such as chocolate or coffee.

Mucilage. A gel-like substance of complex sugar molecules with demulcent and emollient properties; protective of mucous membranes. Flax and quince are mucilaginous.

Narcotic. Numbing, causing stupor, or inducing sleep. Narcotic agents can be addictive.

Nervine. A substance that affects the nervous system; commonly used to refer to something that calms the nerves, but it also may be stimulating. Linden is a nervine with a sedative action.

Nostrum. A favorite but untested remedy; a tonic or patent medicine. Often used to mean a cure-all.

Obstruction. Constipation, kidney stones, or urinary gravel.

Officinal. A drug sold over the counter as a nonprescription medicine; a plant recognized by a pharmacopoeia. Officinal plants include the medicinal rhubarb (*Rheum officinale*), the apothecary rose (*Rosa gallica officinalis*), and the mandrake (*Mandragora officinarum*).

Osteoporosis. Loss of bone density to which menopausal women are especially prone. With the sharp decrease in estrogen at menopause comes a parallel increase in the need for calcium.

Parturition. The act of giving birth.

Patent medicine. A medicine with a patent on its combination of ingredients. In 19th-century America, these medicines were among the first products advertised in publications. Also called tonic or nostrum.

Pectoral. A medicine that is good for the chest; a chest plaster.

Perineum. The pelvic area between the vulva in women (or the scrotum in men) and the anus. In women, perineal tears are common as a result of childbirth. An episiotomy (surgical incision of the perineum) is sometimes performed to facilitate delivery and avoid tearing.

Phlegm. Mucus or sputum.

Physic garden. A medicinal garden.

Piles. Hemorrhoids.

Placenta. The afterbirth.

Plaster. A paste of remedies applied to the chest area, generally at room temperature. See also Poultice.

Pneumonia. A lung infection. Sometimes viral or bacterial; sometimes caused by mucus or other fluids in the lungs.

Posset. Hot milk curdled with alcohol, such as wine or ale, and sweetened, sometimes with other remedies added.

Postpartum. Relating to the first few days after childbirth.

Potherb. Any plant whose leaves, stems, roots, or flowers are cooked and eaten or used as a seasoning. More than 200 years ago, the word *potherb* was the common equivalent of the modern word *vegetable*.

Poultice. A damp mixture of herbs or plant parts (for example, a whole cabbage leaf) applied to the chest or another body part. Generally, the herbs or plant parts are bound between layers of cheesecloth or gauze and kept warm (or hot) and moist.

Premenstrual syndrome (PMS). Emotional and/or physical difficulties before the menses. May include depression, bloating, breast tenderness, constipation or diarrhea, food cravings, or irritability.

Prolapsed uterus. The falling of the womb.

Purgative. Drastically laxative; purging or cleansing.

Receipt book. A recipe book or cookbook; a diary or account book that might contain ongoing records of household accounts along with recipes for cooking and for remedies and other household supplies such as soap and pest repellents.

Reptile. A plant that grows by creeping along the ground. John Lawrence, in *The Clergyman's Recreation* (1726), wrote of "some of those Reptiles useful in the Kitchen viz Carrots, Onions, Parsnips, Spinage, etc."

Resin. A plant substance of clear yellowish or brown color, solid or semisolid and viscous, sometimes used in decocted remedies. The buds of the balm of Gilead, a poplar, are covered with a tacky resin, for example.

Rheumatic fever. A fever and inflammation of the connective tissues.

Rheumatism. A generic term for stiffness and pain in the joints, including arthritis, bursitis, and rheumatic fever.

Rheumatoid arthritis. Chronic and progressive inflammation of the joints. Women are somewhat more prone to it than men.

Rhizome. An underground plant part that grows like a horizontal stem and from which the roots descend. Sometimes decocted and used for remedies.

Rubefacient. Stimulating to the skin and circulation close to the surface of the skin, producing vasodilation (exhibited as reddening) and, in theory, cleansing the affected tissue through increased blood flow. Sometimes called a counter-irritant, such as cayenne pepper, mustard, horseradish, or ginger, and applied for arthritic joints or pleurisy. In the extreme, rubefacients become vesicants, which cause blistering.

Sack. A light, dry, strong wine; sherry.

Sago. A thickener made from the powdery starch of the sago palm.

Salep. A starchy meal made from various Old World orchids and used medicinally as a kind of porridge. See also Sago.

Saleratus. Sodium or potassium bicarbonate, used as a leavening agent much as we use baking soda today. Literally, aerated salt.

Salicin. A bitter glucoside derived from the bark of willows, poplars, and some birches. Aspirin is a synthesized form of salicin.

Saloop. A hot drink made of salep plus sassafras or other aromatic herbs. Also salaup.

Salve. A cream or ointment that can act as a vehicle for herbal remedies.

Saponin. A glycoside that forms a lather, like soap. Soapwort is an example. Some saponins, such as cowslips and mullein, are expectorant; some, such as asparagus, are diuretic. Bile, a natural secretion of the liver, has the effect of saponifying fats to aid digestion.

Scorbutic. Diseased with scurvy.

Scruple. A very small amount; strictly, 20 grains, ⅓ drachm, or ¹⁄₂₄ ounce.

Scurvy. A disease caused by a severe deficiency of vitamin C and exhibited by sore and bleeding gums. Once common among sailors.

Sitz bath. A tub for sitting only, where a therapeutic bath is taken, sometimes using water infused with herbs.

Sleep pillow. A pillow intended to help induce sleep; filled with herbs such as chamomile, dill, hops, lavender, mint, orrisroot, rosemary, sweet marjoram, sweet woodruff, or thyme.

Soporific. Increasing the tendency to sleep. Herbs such as hops have sedative actions and may be considered soporific.

Spirit. The distilled essence of a substance.

Stay. A bag for applying a poultice, such as a chin stay; to stop, as in to stay the menses.

Stitch. A sudden sharp pain or cramp, such as a stitch in the side.

Stone. A hardness or obstruction, such as a kidney stone.

Strep. Streptococcus. A bacterium that can cause an infection anywhere in the body but is commonly known to affect the throat. Symptoms can include fever, sore throat, nasal discharge, difficulty swallowing, lack of appetite, headache, and swollen glands. If followed by a rash, it's considered scarlet fever. Both are commonly treated with antibiotics.

Sudorific. Promoting perspiration.

Sulfur. A pale yellow nonmetallic element sometimes used in remedies (sulfur and molasses for constipation). Also sulphur.

Summer complaint. A summer cold or flu; sometimes diarrhea.

Tannin. A substance usually found in the outer cork, bark, or heartwood of plants, useful in tanning leather. Plants and herbs with tannins are astringent. The more tannin in a plant, the stronger its antiseptic properties. Tannins also tend to be pest repellent.

Tetter. A skin eruption, such as eczema or ringworm.

Tincture. A concentrated solution in which a component of a substance is extracted by means of a solvent; an alcohol solution of a nonvolatile medicine; to stain or tint with a color, as in dyeing. Usually measured in drops. Not to be confused with an infusion or decoction of the same substance, both of which are less concentrated.

Tisane. An herbal infusion, such as barley water or peppermint tea, drunk as a beverage for its mildly medicinal effect. From the Latin *ptisana*, "to crush."

Tonic. A beverage that restores and invigorates; a cleansing beverage meant to help eliminate toxins from the body; sometimes used to mean a patent medicine or nostrum.

Topical. Applied locally, usually to the skin.

Ulcer. A breach in the surface of a membrane or skin.

Unbolted wheat. Bran.

Urethra. The final part of the urinary tract, which runs from the bladder to the outside of the body.

Uterus. The womb.

Volatile. Evaporating readily at normal temperatures.

Volatile oil. A rapidly evaporating oil that does not leave a stain, especially an essential oil. All volatile oils have antiseptic properties.

Wind. Flatulence.

Women's complaint. A gynecological problem, particularly dysmenorrhea.

Wort. From the Old English *wyrt*, meaning "root," "herb," or "plant," as in Saint Johnswort or lungwort.

Further Reading

Erichsen-Brown, Charlotte. *Medicinal and Other Uses of North American Plants: A Historical Survey with Special Reference to the Eastern Indian Tribes.* New York: Dover Publications, Inc., 1979.

Jarvis, DeForest C., M.D. *Folk Medicine.* New York: Holt, Rinehart and Winston, Inc., 1958.

Leighton, Ann. "For Meate or Medicine." *In Early American Gardens.* Boston: Houghton Mifflin Company, 1970.

Lieber, Arnold L. *The Lunar Effect, Biological Tides and Human Emotions.* Garden City, NY: Anchor Press, 1978.

McIntyre, Anne. *The Complete Woman's Herbal: A Manual of Healing Herbs and Nutrition for Personal Well-Being and Family Care.* New York: Henry Holt Company, 1994.

———. *The Herbal for Pregnancy and Childbirth.* Shaftesbury, England: Element Books, Ltd., 1992.

———. *Herbs for Common Ailments.* New York: Simon and Schuster, 1992.

Mills, Simon Y., ed. *The Dictionary of Modern Herbalism: A Comprehensive Guide to Practical Herbal Therapy.* Rochester, VT: Healing Arts Press, 1988.

Ody, Penelope. *The Complete Medicinal Herbal.* New York: Dorling Kindersley, 1993.

————. *Home Herbal: A Practical Guide for Making Herbal Remedies for Common Ailments.* New York: Dorling Kindersley, 1995.

Soule, Deb. *The Roots of Healing.* New York: Citadel Press, 1995.

Weil, Andrew. *Spontaneous Healing.* New York: Alfred A. Knopf, Inc., 1995.

Wesley, John. *Primitive Remedies.* [Originally published as *Primitive Physick,* 1776.] Santa Barbara, CA: Woodbridge Press Publishing Company, 1975.

Worwood, Valerie Ann. *The Fragrant Pharmacy: A Complete Guide to Aromatherapy & Essential Oils.* New York: Bantam Books, 1991.

Index

A

Aaron's rod. *See* great mullein

agrimony, *73*, 116; for **bed-wetting & incontinence**, 73; for **diarrhea or flux**, 67; for **sore throats**, 26

ague tree. *See* sassafras

alehoof. *See* ground ivy

alfalfa, 116; for **menopause**, 87

all-heal. *See* valerian

allium, 116; for **asthma**, 27; for **burns & sunburns**, 43; for **colds**, 25; for **constipation or costiveness**, 69; for **coughs**, 28; for **earache**, 31; for **hair conditioners, rinses & gels**, 105; for **insect bites & stings**, 39; for **insomnia & disturbed sleep**, 109

allspice, 116; for **the menses**, 84; for **toothaches & canker sores**, 43

aloe vera, 116; for **burns & sunburns**, 42, 43; for **hair conditioners, rinses & gels**, 106; for **poison ivy & other itching**, 41

American valerian. *See* lady's slipper

angelica, 116; for **constipation or costiveness**, 70; for **coughs**, 28; for **fever**, 30; for **kidney complaints**, 72; for **the menses**, 84; for **the postpartum period**, 94; for **rheumatism & arthritis**, 37

anise, 116; as **aphrodisiac**, 60; for **coughs**, 28; *To Ease Labor*, 93; for **hiccups**, 45

aphrodisiacs, 60-61

apple, *50, 59, 100; Applesauce Face Mask*, 101; for **asthma**, 27; for **bed-wetting & incontinence**, 73; for **colds**, 59; for **colic**, 59; for **constipation or costiveness**, 59; for **diarrhea or flux**, 59; for **faintings, palpitations & melancholy**, 59; *Mulled Cider*, 59; for **rheumatism**, 59; for **skin afflictions**, 59; for **toothaches & canker sores**, 44; for **urinary tract infections**, 59

arnica, 116-17; for **rheumatism & arthritis**, 38

arthritis, 37-38

artichoke: as **aphrodisiac**, 60; for **kidney complaints**, 72

asparagus: for **kidney complaints**, 72

asthma, 27

B

backwort. *See* comfrey

balm of Gilead, 117; for **menopause**, 87

balsam: for **coughs**, 28; for **poison ivy &**